BODY HEAT

WARNING

BODY HEAT

Andrew Nash
with
Alaistair Crommelin

Foreword by
Sally Gunnell MBE

B⊞XTREE

First published in Great Britain in 1996 by Boxtree Limited

Text © Boxtree 1996
Illustrations © Catherine Ward 1996

Body Heat was created by Stephen Leahy and is an Action Time Production with Carlton UK Productions.

©Carlton UK Television Limited MCMXCVI

Designed by K DESIGN, Winscombe, Somerset
Printed and bound in the UK by Bath Press, Somerset for

Boxtree Limited
Broadwall House
21 Broadwall
London SE1 9PL

A CIP catalogue entry for this book is available from the British Library.

ISBN 0 7522 1089 0

Cover photographs by John Rogers © John Rogers/Carlton Television

CONTENTS

SALLY GUNNELL MBE

Body Heat is one of the highlights of my year. And not just because it's not me having to work hard for a change! For the last three years I have spent several enjoyable weeks watching competitors fight their way through the heats, and seen them sweat under the studio lights trying to achieve a place in the final.

My co-presenter, Jeremy Guscott, and I love the time we have spent getting to know the finalists in Atlanta, Georgia and South Africa. Seeing their dedication helps remind us of how hard we must train to win on the track or the rugby field.

When I was first asked to become one of the presenters on Body Heat I was thrilled by the prospect. It was a great opportunity to do something different and exciting – behind the camera for a change – but most importantly it was to do with sport. I love all that competition and I get a great buzz out of presenting the programme and watching people really push themselves.

Once the show starts I find myself getting goose bumps all over, feeling all the emotions I have myself before I compete. More than anyone else there, Jeremy and I know what the competitors are putting themselves through. I know how hard they have trained; I know what they have been through to get there. When I am watching the competitors driving themselves to exhaustion on the endurance test or the bleep test I find myself cheering them on and thinking 'these people really are fit' as well as 'I'm glad I don't have to do that!'

It's difficult not to get emotionally involved during the recordings and sometimes I wonder how the competitors cope. What amazes me is that it is not a one-off event – one race and that's it. They have to do three different events in one evening: the endurance test, the bleep test and the grand finale of the tri batak. Body Heat is about people pushing themselves to a limit and then having to recover and go out and do it again. For me it would be like running a heat, a semi-final and a final all in one day, having to improve my performance each time.

You cannot compare Body Heat to other TV shows because it has different demands. It is not just about sheer muscular strength but also involves power, endurance and the ability to think fast under pressure. It is the ultimate in cross training and I have to admit that if I went out to compete on Body Heat I would not be very good at all the events. The other competitors would beat me into the ground on quite a lot of it, though I'd definitely fancy my chances in the sprint relay!

What I do is very specialist; I'm always training for one specific event – the 400 metre hurdles – whereas in Body Heat they are training for general fitness and need to excel in everything. If I went on a bike I'd be useless, as it uses totally different muscles. The step machines, the bikes, the endurance event are all very different from what I am used to doing. I've only tried the bleep test once and that was enough. I did it as part of a training session, but I had already trained that morning and so I only went up to Level 11 – which is not very high at all – but that gave me an idea of how hard it is. Now every time I see other people doing it I'm very happy I don't have to!

Although it looks very different there is a direct connection between what I do at the Olympics or the World Championships and what the Body Heat competitors do. We are all aiming to win. My whole life comes down to a single race on a particular day. It is a race that lasts under 54 seconds but everything I do is geared towards its outcome. The setting may be different but, like me, Body Heat competitors have been in very serious training for six months and it has been their life as it has for me. They have trained really hard for their one chance in a Nottingham TV studio.

There are days when the weather is awful and I don't want to go training but deep down I know I have to. What will I achieve if I don't do it when my rivals and competitors are out there hurting? There is nothing you can do in training, however, that will prepare you for a race or for running in front of a crowd. I can always see how Body Heat competitors are all very, very, nervous before they start; some people love having others cheer them on, others don't. After years of competing I have got used to that side of things but I can still remember how I used to feel.

As an athlete I am naturally aware of how important it is to be physically fit. Every year when I present Body Heat it reminds me of how hard ordinary men and women, teachers, policemen and mothers have worked to be there, juggling their jobs and their families to train and compete. None of the competitors I've spoken to have ever regretted a moment of all that hard work.

Hopefully this book is a way for everybody to share in our experience, and to get fit and healthy. Following the authors' exercise plan and diet guidelines will make a new woman or man out of you in six months. Rest assured it's not all hard work being fit – one of the best things is knowing that you can have a beer and a chocolate bar without feeling guilty. I look forward to seeing some of you competing – and winning – in Body Heat in the years ahead.

One day in the future I'm going to retire from athletics, though I hope I'll still be presenting Body Heat for many years to come. When I finish I'm still going to keep myself fit and

I'd like to do more cross training, like swimming, biking and playing tennis. So in some ways I may well end up better equipped and fitter to do Body Heat than I am now. But I doubt I'll ever want to do that bleep test again!

Sally Gunnell

CHAPTER 1

WELCOME TO BODY HEAT

Inside the TV studio the noise is deafening, cheers and yells driving the six Lycra-clad bodies on to greater and greater effort. But the competitors hear little of this for they are pushing themselves on, faster, harder, feet catapulting off the board, back and shoulders taking the strain, then the arms pulling the stroke through. No one is going anywhere for the rowing machines do not move and the immense effort the three men and three women are expelling is being registered by a computer.

The competitors do not care, they are pumped up, giving their all, determined to beat their two rivals, willing their partner to do the same to her rivals. At stake is more than just pride. This is the culmination of months, perhaps years of hard training. Much of that was done in private but this is very much in public. This is real, this is on television. This is Body Heat.

For the past three years millions of people have watched Body Heat, the Carlton Television series presented by Mike Smith with Olympic 400 metre hurdles champion Sally Gunnell, and England Rugby Union centre Jeremy Guscott. It is a programme in which ordinary couples from all over Britain try to prove themselves champions. Police officers, fitness instructors, merchant bankers, market traders, bank managers, sales reps, students, actors, models, aerobics instructors, stock brokers, servicemen, housewives and mothers have all shown their commitment and given 110% in an attempt to show they are fitter than their rivals.

On the telly it never seems that tough. After all, what's so difficult about the Endurance Test, cycling 4000 metres in under 10 minutes, or running a 2 × 200 metre relay? There's something called the 'bleep test' which makes all the competitors blood run pale. It can't be that hard to just keep jogging a bit faster very time the bleep goes, can it? If you're sitting at home in your armchair guzzling a beer, it's not hard at all. However, if you are out there and the pace keeps speeding up and up and your closest rival is still going strong and your breathing is getting shallower and shallower and your legs feel like lead, getting heavier with every step, then it's really, really hard.

In fact, if it looks that easy on the telly why don't you have a go? Yes, you in the armchair. The one who has been talking for months about how you would like to get properly fit, losing some of that weight you put on at Christmas and never got round to taking off. You could be on Body Heat if you wanted. It won't be easy, in fact it'll be downright tough, but you can do it. Just keep reading.

In the next 16 chapters we have designed an exercise programme which over the next six months will take an unfit man or woman to a level of physical fitness at which they could audition for the next series of Body Heat and not embarrass themselves.

Andrew Nash, who was a finalist in the first ever series of Body Heat but now works as the fitness consultant to the TV series, has designed a graduated exercise programme. It starts with brisk walks around the local park, stresses the importance of warming up and stretching, guides you through the pitfalls of choosing a gym and how to operate the fitness machines, and culminates in a regular full-body workout in the gym. Along the way your body will tighten up, muscles become taut and toned. At the end you will be able to feel justifiably proud.

Sally Gunnell and Jeremy Guscott have provided us with some tips and advice that may sound simple but, believe us, are the product of hard-won experience and years of training. You don't get to the top of your profession without expending a lot of sweat and a few tears.

The two chapters on Body Food are designed to introduce you to the possibilities of changing your diet and eating habits to help cope with the new demands that fitness will place on your body. We try to explain why certain foods are better for you than others and, by giving examples of low calorie meals and menu plans, enable even the most ham-fisted cook to prepare nutritious and tasty meals.

In the final part of the book you will learn how to prepare for taking part in Body Heat. There is a special training programme designed to bring you to peak fitness in time for the auditions and advice on how to tackle the tests on the show. 1995 finalist Kirstie Chapman recounts what happened when she decided to go for it, while past winners and finalists have kindly provided us with their training schedules so you can learn how to adapt their regime to your specific needs. And finally we give you some tips on how to psyche yourself up to win.

See you in the Body Heat Final soon.

CHAPTER 2

UNDERSTANDING YOUR BODY

Your decision to carry out a physical fitness programme is not one to be taken lightly. It requires a lifelong commitment of time and effort. Exercise must become one of those things that you do without question, like bathing and brushing your teeth. Patience is essential. Don't try to do too much too soon and don't quit before you have a chance to experience the rewards of improved fitness. You can't regain in a few days or weeks what you have lost in years of sedentary living, but you can get it back If you persevere. And the prize is worth the price.

It may sound as if we are being pernickety, but if you are to become seriously fit, you need to understand a great deal about how the body works. If you understand some of the basic physiology it will help you avoid injury or over-exertion later on. And if you are really getting into training there is nothing worse than suddenly being laid up with a niggle or a muscle strain you could have avoided. The chapters on Stretching and Body Food also contain medical and physiological information that may be of use.

COMPONENTS OF PHYSICAL FITNESS

Physical fitness is to the human body what fine tuning is to an engine. It enables us to perform to our potential. Fitness can be described as a condition that helps us look, feel and do our best. It is: The ability to perform daily tasks vigorously and alertly, with energy left over for enjoying leisure-time activities and meeting emergency demands. It is the ability to endure, to bear up, to withstand stress, to carry on in circumstances where an unfit person could not continue, and is a major basis for good health and well-being.

Physical fitness involves the performance of the heart and lungs, and the muscles of the body. And, since what we do with our bodies also affects what we can do with our minds, fitness influences to some degree qualities such as mental alertness and emotional stability. As you undertake your fitness programme, it's important to remember that fitness is an individual quality that varies from person to person. It is influenced by age, sex, heredity, personal habits, exercise and eating practices. You can't do anything about the first three factors. However, it is within your power to change and improve the others where needed.

Physical fitness is most easily understood by examining its different constituent parts. There are four basic components:

Cardiorespiratory (or Cardiovascular) Endurance – the ability to deliver oxygen and nutrients to tissues, and to remove waste products over sustained periods of time. Long runs and swims are among the methods employed in measuring this component. In the Body Heat TV series this is measured by the various endurance tests which push the body to the limit.

Muscular Strength – the ability of a muscle to exert force over a period of time. Upper-body strength, for example, can be measured by various weight-lifting exercises. In Body Heat it is measured by the Cybex machines.

Muscular Endurance – the ability of a muscle, or a group of muscles, to sustain repeated contractions or to continue applying force against a fixed object. Press-ups are often used to test endurance of arm and shoulder muscles. In Body Heat this is measured by both the Cybex machine and by the endurance exercises.

Flexibility – the ability to move joints and use muscles through their full range of motion. The sit-and-reach test is a good measure of flexibility of the lower back and backs of the upper legs. Although this is not tested on the TV programme (it is very difficult to devise a competitive flexibility test – you're either flexible or you're not) it is not something we ignore in our exercise programme.

Body Composition – often considered a component of fitness, it refers to the makeup of the body in terms of lean body mass (muscle, bone, vital tissue and organs) and fat mass. An optimal ratio of fat to lean mass is an indication of fitness, and the right types of exercise will help you decrease body fat, and increase or maintain muscle mass.

To these four we would like to add:

Mental Alertness – but, you say, mental alertness or agility is not related to physical fitness. No, you can't do brain press ups and cerebral squats, but regular physical exercise should have a beneficial effect on your thought processes by increasing alertness. Throughout the exercise programme we encourage variety as this in turn encourages the brain to keep working. If you have seen the Body Heat TV show you know that mental agility plays an important part, whether it be in answering questions, or tackling problems dangling on a rope during Pressure Points, or simply having the mental strength to keep your body coordinated during the last onslaught of the Tri Batak.

KNOWING YOUR BODY

PULSE RATES

To be fit for Body Heat you have to be aerobically fit. This involves working for long periods of time with your body at between 60% and 85% of your Maximum Heart Rate. Many gym machines have pulse monitors and require you to feed information in to get the correct results so it might help to know what we're talking about.

There are three pulse rates to be aware of, and it takes practise to learn how to measure pulse rates correctly so, before starting the Body Heat programme, spend a week monitoring your pulse at different times of the day .

Your pulse may be found either at the main artery on the side of your neck, just below the junction of the jaw, or on the flat side of your wrist in line with your thumb. You may take your pulse at the base of the neck by pressing lightly on the carotid artery located to the left or right of your Adam's apple. However, too much pressure placed on the carotid artery may stimulate a reflex mechanism that causes the heart to slow down. A more accurate place to count the pulse is at the wrist. Simply press with the first two fingers of one hand and count the number of beats. It is more accurate to take the pulse over a full minute though if rushed you can take it for 15 seconds and multiply by 4, or even 10 seconds and multiply by 6.

1. RESTING PULSE RATE

The ideal time to find your true resting heart rate is in the morning, after a good night's sleep before you get out of bed. Count your pulse for one whole minute to find your resting heart rate. Do this for three days and take the average as your resting rate. In the future if the rate is over 10 bpm (beats per minute) higher than that average, do not train during the day as you are too tired or perhaps even ill.

2. MAXIMUM HEART RATE

Simply deduct your age in years from 220. This is approximately your MHR – the maximum amount your heart can beat in a minute. Above that you are pushing yourself too hard and depriving the blood of oxygen. For example, the MHR of a 20-year-old woman is 200, while for a 35-year-old man it is 185.

3. TARGET HEART RATE ZONE

Your aim is to get your heart beating, pumping oxygen around the body as efficiently as possible. First it is necessary to calculate your target heart rate zone, which will give you both a minimum and a maximum exercise heart rate. The simplest rule of thumb is to make sure that your heart exercise rate varies between 60–85% of your Maximum Heart Rate. If you do not achieve this level for more than 20 minutes of an exercise session at least three times a week you are not actually increasing your training capability, merely standing still. However at the beginning of your exercise schedule you should not work at levels above 75% MHR as this can be counter-productive.

BODY SHAPE AND PHYSIQUE

Look around any gym and you will soon see that people have a certain fundamental shape that they cannot change. The three standard body type classifications are:

Ectomorph – long and lean with narrow shoulders and hips, relatively long legs and arms, narrow fingers and toes and a delicate bone structure. Ectomorphs make good long-distance runners, but can have problems carrying weight over distance.

Mesomorph – strong, energetic and muscular with broad shoulders and narrow hips, heavy bone and muscle development, broad hands and a muscular chest. Mesomorphs make good weight-lifters and swimmers.

Endomorph – round and soft, with wide hips, round faces, often with slender wrists and ankles and relatively small facial features. Endomorphs have the problem that they can gain weight easily and even when not overweight look rounded . . . and cuddly.

Naturally it is not as simple as that. Many people are in fact a combination of different classifications and a careful regime of diet and exercise might change the balance between the two.

Body shapes can also be classified into four categories:

The Pear – narrow shoulders, a small chest, average waist, and wider hips and buttocks. Fat is usually concentrated in the hips and thighs.

The Box – often looks straight up and down with no visible waistline. Fat is usually concentrated in the waist.

The Inverted Triangle – broad shoulders and narrow hips. Fat is usually concentrated in the chest.

The Hourglass Figure – broad hips and chest and a small waist. Fat is usually concentrated in the chest and hips.

Look in a mirror and you will know what you are. That is your genetic inheritance. If you are a woman with a small bust and large thighs (a pear) you cannot change into a Marilyn Monroe (Hourglass figure) without resorting to surgery. What you can do is tone your body so that your pectoral, abdominal and gluteal (bottom) muscles develop, and the fat deposits in the hips and thighs diminish to become much sleeker and more aesthetically pleasing. You can improve or make the very best of that genetic inheritance just like you can improve your muscular strength, the amount of oxygen your lungs can process, and your endurance. But you cannot change it. Accept that and aim to improve it instead.

You can be overweight without being over fat. Or, you could be over fat without being overweight. Excess fat is a health concern, not excess weight. For example, a Rugby lock forward may weigh 17 stone (238lbs) and according to standard height/weight charts, he is overweight. But this person's 'excess' weight is due to lots of muscle mass and large, dense bones. So, when assessing your overall fitness, it's the percentage of your body that is composed of fat, and not your weight in itself, that makes the difference.

However, there is one thing to be aware of: while all body types can be improved there is a finite level of improvement which we all have to accept. The commonly held view at present is that physical ability is 75% genetic and 25% training and environment.

When we talk about body 'fat' we mean the percentage of your body weight that is made up of fat. Males and females have different body composition. The average male is 6in taller and heavier and when fit should comprise 42% muscle, 12–14% body fat and carries 4% more water. The average female should have 36% muscle and 20–25% fat.

All of us require some stored body fat for fuelling energy – if the body has too little fat, it will begin to break down muscle tissue for energy requirements. Some female athletes, particularly distance runners, have so little body fat that it can have other effects on the body. For example, menstrual cycles can become irregular or cease altogether.

MEASURING BODY FAT

Percent body fat (the percentage of the body that is composed of fat) can be determined by measuring the thickness of sub-cutaneous fat at various locations on the body. The measurements obtained are used in special equations to obtain an estimated percent fat value. Many gyms offer an accurate reading taken either by skin-fold callipers which are used to measure the fat below the skin's surface, or electronic machines.

If you want to do it at home try the pinch test. Take a pinch of flesh between thumb and forefinger in the following four places: biceps (upper arms, front), triceps (upper arm, back) sub-scapular (beneath the shoulder blade), suprailiac (one inch above and along from the hip bone). Make a note of how much flesh you can pinch and you will be able to compare how you are getting along. It's only approximate but it's easy.

TO WEIGH OR NOT TO WEIGH

There are serious pitfalls in relying on the bathroom scales. By looking at a standardized height/weight chart, you can determine if you weigh more (overweight) or less (underweight) than the average person with a height and frame size similar to your height and frame size. A height/weight chart cannot be used to determine if you are 'over fat'. Therefore, weighing yourself on a scale tells you very little about your health.

Remember that a scale tells you only how much you weigh.

That's all it tells you. It measures not only your body fat but also any muscle gain, water, food, and anything else hanging around in your intestines. Similarly, weighing yourself after a hard workout may reveal you have lost 5lb. Yes, 5lb of sweat that will be replaced the moment you finish drinking. If you insist on weighing yourself the only time to do it is first thing in the morning. Get up, empty your bladder and then step onto the scales before you consume anything else. That is your body weight pure and unadulterated. If you wish to keep a record keep doing it at the same time so there is a valid comparison. But remember one thing: muscle weighs more than fat so as you become fitter you may even put on weight. Don't break the scales, it's not their fault!

PRE-EXERCISE MEDICAL QUESTIONNAIRE

Before starting the programme please answer the following questions with either Yes or No:

1. Has your doctor ever said you have heart disease, high blood pressure or any other cardiovascular problem?
2. Is there a history of heart disease in your family?
3. Has your doctor ever said you have high blood pressure?
4. Do you ever have pains in your heart and chest, after undergoing minimal exertion?
5. Do you often get headaches, feel faint or dizzy?
6. Do you suffer from pain or limited movement in any joints or bones which has either been aggravated by exercise or might might be made worse by it?
7. Are you taking drugs or medication or recuperating from a recent illness or operation at the moment?
8. Are you pregnant?
9. Do you have any other condition which might affect your ability to participate in exercise?
10. Are you over 35 and unaccustomed to physical exercise?

If you answered YES to one or more questions consult your

doctor *before* starting the programme and ask his advice as to whether you can undertake unrestricted physical training/activity on a gradually increasing basis. If he suggests only restricted or supervized activities for an initial period, discuss whether Body Heat Programme will fulfil these criteria.

If you answered NO to all questions you should feel reasonably assured that you are a suitable case for exercise. However, if you have a temporary illness, even a minor cold a cough or a slight sore throat, postpone starting the programme until you are fully recovered and ready to hit the ground running.

SALLY'S TIPS

Now you are ready to start, here are Sally Gunnell's tips on how to get the most from your training.

1. Remember, quality is the key to training and competition.
2. Look after your body by warming up and down properly – I spend one hour before a race warming up.
3. Treat any injury problems immediately.
4. Try and train with a group of friends – sport is better fun together.
5. Set realistic goals for yourself.
6. Be motivated and patient, but also keep at it – results take time.
7. Whatever sport you do, flexibility is very important to achieve your best results.
8. Drink plenty of water to replace lost fluids during heavy exercise. I drink 6–8 glasses of water a day.
9. Don't eat two hours before doing any exercise – you can get a bad attack of stitch and sometimes feel sick which will not help you win anything.
10. I eat a varied but healthy diet – lots of fruit and vegetables. I get protein from chicken and fish, carbohydrates from rice and pasta. Remember, not too much fat and sugar.
11. Shoes are the most important part of your training equipment. These need to be supportive, have good cushioning and obviously fit correctly.
12. Badly worn shoes can cause injury.
13. Don't be tempted to take drugs to enhance your performance. You can easily damage your health.
14. Stay clear of high sugar drinks. They will give you a boost in the short term but they really don't do you any good.
15. Keep a record of your exercise regime on a day-to-day basis. It's encouraging to watch your progress and it also helps to highlight the parts that may not be working for you.

CHAPTER 3

BODY WARM: STRETCHING, WARM-UPS AND COOL DOWNS

It is impossible to over-stress the importance of stretching before taking part in any kind of exercise. The older you get the more important it becomes, as the muscles start to lose the elasticity of youth. Before each race Sally Gunnell will spend up to an hour warming up, stretching and preparing for an event which lasts less than a minute. We're not suggesting that you apply Olympian standards, but warming up and stretching must become an integral part of your training schedule. You should always allow 10 minutes for warming up at the beginning and a further 5 minutes at the end to cool down.

The reasons for this are two-fold. Proper preparation cuts down the risk of injury by making sure your muscles are warmed up and ready. Secondly, good and regular stretching increases the body's flexibility which is one of the major components of physical fitness. Just because it is often ignored (primarily by male athletes) does not mean it is not important. Nobody is expecting you to be able to turn yourself inside out like a gymnast but it's pretty embarrassing not to be able to touch your toes.

JEREMY'S TRAINING TIP
WARMING UP

Until a couple of years ago rugby training was a very old-fashioned thing. We used to run out on the training pitch, play a game of touch rugby, run around at a hundred miles an hour, pulling, straining and tearing everything before we even started. Whereas an athlete like Sally was taught from the word go to warm up properly. Now we spend literally 30 to 45 minutes with our fitness conditioner stretching and warming up the big muscle groups to get us to run at 100% and prepare our bodies for contact. The warm-up has become the most important part of our training alongside the warming down – that is also essential. If you walk straight off the paddock without warming down you will get stiff and can do yourself some damage.

I never worked on getting myself supple, bending, touching my toes. Now the more injuries I pick up, the more I look to warming up. Two years ago I had a year out through injury, a deep-seated groin strain that would not go away. I'm sure it was wear and tear and if I had been educated in the way of warming up properly, if I had looked after myself properly, it might never have occurred.

WHY YOU NEED TO STRETCH

At the risk of getting rather technical, let's have a quick look at how muscles work. Taken together, muscles and bones make up the musculo-skeletal system of the body. The bones provide posture and structural support for the body, while the muscles provide the body with its ability to move. The musculo-skeletal system also provides protection for the body's internal organs. In order to serve their function, bones must be joined together by something. The point where bones connect to one another is called a joint, and this connection is made mostly by ligaments helped by muscles. Muscles are attached to the bone by tendons. Bones, tendons, and ligaments cannot make your body move. Only muscles can.

Muscles vary in shape and in size, and serve many different purposes. Most large muscles, like the hamstrings and quadri-

15

ceps in the legs, and the biceps and triceps in the upper arms, control motion. Others, like the heart and the muscles of the inner ear, perform other equally vital functions. At the microscopic level, however, all muscles share the same basic structure.

The whole muscle is composed of bundles of tissue called fasciculi. These are the strands of muscle that we see when we cut into a steak or a chicken leg. Each fasciculus is composed of bundles of muscle fibres. The muscle fibres are in turn composed of tens of thousands of thread-like myofybrils, which can each contract, relax, and lengthen. The myofybrils are composed of up to millions of bands laid end-to-end called sarcomeres. Each sarcomere is made of overlapping thick and thin filaments called myofilaments.

Muscles work when they receive an electrical signal transmitted from the brain via the spinal column to the nerves. The nerve and muscle connect at the neuromuscular junction. When an electrical signal crosses the neuromuscular junction, it is transmitted deep inside the muscle fibres where the signal stimulates the flow of calcium which causes the thick and thin myofilaments to slide across one another. This causes the sarcomere to shorten, which generates force. When billions of sarcomeres in the muscle shorten all at once this results in a contraction of the entire muscle fibre. When a muscle fibre contracts, it contracts completely. If the force of the muscle contraction needs to be stronger more muscle fibres are recruited to perform the job. The more muscle fibres recruited by the central nervous system, the stronger the force generated by the muscular contraction. In other words, the more you work your muscles, the stronger they become.

Located all around the muscle and its fibres are connective tissues. Connective tissue is composed of a base substance and two kinds of protein-based fibre – collagenous connective tissue and elastic connective tissue. Collagenous connective tissue consists mostly of collagen and provides tensile strength. Elastic connective tissue consists mostly of elastin and provides elasticity. The base substance is called mucopolysaccharide and is altogether pretty smart. It acts as both a lubricant, allowing the fibres to slide easily over one another, and as a glue, holding the fibres of the tissue together into bundles. The more elastic connective tissue there is around a joint, the greater the range of motion in that joint. Connective tissues are made up of tendons, ligaments, and the fascial sheaths that envelop, or bind down, muscles into separate groups.

When you stretch a muscle fibre, the sarcomere stretches and the area of overlap between the thick and thin myofilaments decreases, allowing the muscle fibre to elongate. Once all the sarcomeres are fully stretched, additional stretching places force on the surrounding connective tissue. As the tension increases, the collagen fibres in the connective tissue align themselves along the same line of force as the tension. Hence when you stretch, the muscle fibre is pulled out to its full length, sarcomere by sarcomere, and the connective tissue takes up the remaining slack. When this occurs, it helps to realign any disorganized fibres in the direction of the tension. (This realignment is what helps to rehabilitate scarred tissue back to health.)

Just as the total strength of a contracting muscle is a result of the number of fibres contracting, the total length of a stretched muscle is a result of the number of fibres stretched – the more fibres stretched, the more length developed by the muscle for a given stretch. The more fibres used in a stretch, the more fibres there are standing by to contract and provide force when next you need them. From a physiological point of view, stretching is good for you !

How to Stretch

When done properly, stretching can do more than just increase flexibility. The benefits of stretching include:

- increased mental and physical relaxation
- enhanced development of body awareness

- reduced risk of injury to joints, muscles and tendons
- reduced muscular soreness
- reduced muscular tension

Unfortunately, even those who stretch do not always stretch properly and hence do not reap some or all of these benefits. Some of the most common mistakes made when stretching are:

- improper warm-up
- inadequate rest between workouts
- overstretching
- performing the wrong exercises
- performing exercises in the wrong (or sub-optimal) sequence

In this chapter, we will try to show you how to avoid these problems, and others, and present some of the most effective methods for realizing all the benefits of stretching.

WARMING UP

Stretching is not warming up! It is, however, a very important, essential, part of warming up. Warming up is exactly what it says – the process of raising your core body temperature by one or two degrees Celsius (1.4 to 2.8 degrees Fahrenheit).

A warm up is divided into three parts – general warm up, stretching, and sport-specific activity. It is not a good idea to attempt to stretch before your muscles are warm. Warming up can do more than just loosen stiff muscles; when done properly, it can actually improve performance. On the other hand, an improper warm-up, or no warm-up at all, can greatly increase your risk of injury. The goals of the warm-up are an increased awareness, improved coordination, improved elasticity and contractibility of muscles, and a greater efficiency of the respiratory and cardiovascular systems.

GENERAL WARM-UP

The general warm-up is divided into two parts: joint rotations and aerobic activity. These two activities should be performed in the right order.

The general warm-up should begin with joint rotations. Start either from your toes and work your way up, or from your fingers (hands above head) and work your way down. This lubricates your joints with synovial fluid, permits them to function more easily and increases mobility. The whole body should be relaxed and you should perform slow circular movements, both clockwise and counter-clockwise, until the joint seems to move smoothly. Do not jerk and do not push the head back when rotating the neck. It may seem a lot to do but should only take 3–4 minutes.

Rotate the following (in the order given, or in the reverse order):

1. Fingers and knuckles
2. Wrists
3. Elbows
4. Shoulders
5. Neck
6. Trunk/waist
7. Hips
8. Legs
9. Knees
10. Ankles
11. Toes

After you have performed the joint rotations, you should engage in at least five minutes of aerobic activity such as jogging on the spot, knee raises, bum kicks (kicking heel up to touch backside), side touches (stepping from side to side), pushing arms above the head or punching in front, skipping, or any other activity that will get your blood pumping round the body. The purpose of this is to raise your core body temperature and get your blood flowing. Increased blood flow in the muscles improves muscle performance and flexibility and reduces the likelihood of injury.

WARM-UP STRETCHING

Once the general warm-up has been completed, the muscles are warmer and more elastic. Immediately following your general warm-up, you should engage in some slow, relaxed, static stretching. You should start with your back, followed by your upper body and lower body, stretching your muscles in the order listed below. Unfortunately, not everyone has the time to stretch all their muscles before a workout. At least take the time to stretch all the muscles that will be heavily used during your workout.

Many people are unaware of the fact that the order in which you perform your stretching exercises is important. Often, when we perform a particular stretch, it actually stretches more than one group of muscles – the muscles that the stretch is primarily intended for, and other supporting muscles that are also stretched but which do not receive the 'brunt' of the stretch. These supporting muscles usually function as synergists for the muscles being stretched. Before performing a stretch intended for a particular muscle, but which actually stretches several muscles, you should first stretch each of that muscle's synergists. The benefit of this is that you can stretch the primary muscles better by not allowing the supporting muscles the opportunity to be a limiting factor in how 'good' a stretch you can attain for a particular exercise.

Ideally, it is best to perform a stretch that isolates a particular muscle group, but this is not always possible. By organizing the exercises within a stretching routine according to the principle of interdependency of muscle groups, you minimize the effort required to perform the routine, and maximize the effectiveness of the individual exercises.

For example, a stretch intended primarily for the hamstrings may also make some demands upon the calves and bum (and even the lower back) but mostly, it stretches the hamstrings. In this case, it would be a good idea to stretch the lower back, backside, and calves first (in that order, using stretches intended primarily for those muscles) before they need to be used in a stretch that is intended primarily for the hamstrings.

As a general rule, you should usually do the following when putting together a stretching routine:

- stretch your back (upper and lower) first
- stretch your sides after stretching your back
- stretch your buttocks before stretching your groin or your hamstrings
- stretch your calves before stretching your hamstrings
- stretch your shins before stretching your quadriceps (if you do shin stretches)
- stretch your arms before stretching your chest

This is the order in which you should carry out your stretching routine. At the end of the chapter you will find a series of stretches which apply to each of these muscle groups:

1. Back
2. Sides (external obliques)
3. Shoulders
4. Triceps
5. Chest
6. Buttocks
7. Groin (adductors)
8. Hips
9. Thighs (quadriceps and abductors)
10. Calves
11. Hamstrings

SPORT-SPECIFIC ACTIVITY

The last part of your warm-up should be devoted to performing movements that mirror the movements that you will be performing during your athletic activity, rehearsing specific movements that the athlete will be using during the practise or the event, but at a reduced intensity. Sport-specific activities improve coordination, balance, strength, and response time, and may reduce the risk of injury.

COOLING DOWN

Stretching is only part of the process of cooling down, not the be all and end all. After you have completed your workout, the best way to reduce muscle fatigue and soreness – which is caused by the lactic acid produced in the muscles as a waste by-product of your exertions – is to perform a light warm-down. This warm-down is similar to the second half of your warm-up (but in the reverse order) and consists of two phases: light aerobic/sport-specific activity and static stretching.

Ideally, you should start your warm-down with about 10–20 mins of sport-specific activity but that is usually unrealistic in these time-tight days. You should, however, attempt to perform at least 5 mins of sport-specific activity at a lower intensity than that of your workout. This should immediately be followed by some relaxed, static stretches which can reduce cramping, tightening, and soreness in fatigued muscles and will make you feel better. A light warm-down exercise immediately following maximal exertion is a better way of clearing lactic acid from the blood than complete rest. Furthermore, if you are still sore the next day, a light warm-down is a good way to reduce lingering muscle tightness and soreness even when not performed immediately after a workout.

HOW LONG SHOULD I HOLD A STRETCH FOR?

Good question. Expert opinion varies from as little as 10 seconds to several minutes. Recent research on the hamstring stretches indicates that 15 seconds may be sufficient, but whether that may be sufficient for other muscle groups is unclear. Let's compromise on an average 15–20 secs during warm-up and 20–30 secs during cool down. (Children, and adolescents whose bones are still growing, do not need to hold a passive stretch this long – 7–10 secs would be fine.) Remember it is better to stretch a little than not at all, so if you are pushed for time make sure you can stretch both before and after exercise. On the other hand if you are in no hurry it is a very good idea to perform your stretches in sets of 2–5 repetitions with a 15–30 second rest in between each stretch. If you don't have a watch handy it's a good idea to count during the duration of the stretch.

Proper breathing helps to relax the body, increases blood flow throughout the body, and helps to mechanically remove lactic acid and other by-products of exercise. Take slow, relaxed breaths when you stretch, trying to exhale as the muscle is stretching. Some experts even recommend increasing the intensity of the stretch only while exhaling, holding the stretch in its current position at all other times. Inhale slowly through the nose, expanding the abdomen (not the chest); hold the breath a moment; then exhale slowly through the mouth. Inhaling through the nose has several purposes including cleaning the air and ensuring proper temperature and humidity for oxygen transfer into the lungs. The rate of breathing should be controlled through the use of the glottis in the back of the throat. This produces a very soft 'hm-m-m-mn' sound inside the throat as opposed to a sniffing sound in the sinuses. The exhalation should be controlled in a similar manner but with more of an 'ah-h-h-h-h' sound, like the sigh of relief you feel at having survived another session.

As you breathe in, the diaphragm presses downward on the internal organs and their associated blood vessels, squeezing the blood out of them. As you exhale, the abdomen, its organs and muscles, and their blood vessels flood with new blood. This rhythmic contraction and expansion of the abdominal blood vessels is partially responsible for the circulation of blood in the body. Also, the rhythmic pumping action helps to remove waste products from the muscles in the torso. This pumping action is referred to as the respiratory pump.

WHEN TO STRETCH

It is advisable to stretch at least once a day, even when you are not planning on taking any other exercise. Most of us know what it is like for two days after the first cricket, football or tennis game of the year – stiffness and sometimes agony as muscles not used for ages make themselves felt and stretching will help alleviate this. And for the exercises to be of proper benefit, you must perform them correctly every day. So make a habit of stretching for a minimum of 10 minutes every day. The best time to stretch is when your muscles are warmed up. If they are not already warm before you wish to stretch, then you need to warm them up yourself, usually by performing some type of brief aerobic activity. If the weather is very cold, or if you are feeling very stiff, then you need to take extra care to warm-up before you stretch in order to reduce the risk of injuring yourself.

Everyone has their own internal body-clock, or circadian rhythm as the scientists have christened it. Some of us are early morning people while others are night owls. Being aware of your circadian rhythm should help you decide when it is best for you to exercise (or indeed perform any other type of activity). Research indicates that most people are more flexible in the afternoon than in the morning, peaking from about 2:30pm – 4pm and that flexibility and strength are greatest in the late afternoon or early evening. If this is true, then an athlete might get a better workout by hitting the gym right after work rather than before it. The best judge of all this is – as always – you. It's your body and you understand its rhythms. Once you are taking on regular exercise programme a combination of social and physical factors will determine when you take that exercise. Listen to your body, it generally knows best.

PAIN AND DISCOMFORT

Your body certainly knows best if you are experiencing any pain. Unfortunately, a certain amount of muscular soreness, pain, discomfort and even injury are part of the athlete's lot. If you are experiencing pain or discomfort before, during, or after stretching or athletic activity, then you need to try to identify the cause. Severe pain (particularly in the joints, ligaments, or tendons) usually indicates a serious injury of some sort, and you may need to stop exercising until you have recovered. If in doubt always seek medical advice.

If you are experiencing soreness, stiffness, or some other form of muscular pain, then it may be due to a torn tissue. Overstretching and engaging in athletic activities without a proper warm-up can cause microscopic tearing of muscle fibres or connective tissues. If the tear is not too severe, the pain will usually not appear until one or two days after the activity that caused the damage. If the pain occurs during or immediately after the activity, then it may indicate a more serious tear which may require immediate medical attention. If the pain is not too severe, then it is permissable to perform light, careful static stretching of the injured area under professional supervision. Torn fibres heal at a shortened length which decreases flexibility in the injured muscles. Very light stretching of the injured muscles helps reduce loss of flexibility resulting from the injury. Intense stretching of any kind, however, may only make matters worse.

Overexertion and/or intense muscular activity will fatigue the muscles and cause them to accumulate lactic acid and other waste products. If this is the cause of your pain, then stretching, and a good cool down (see p.22 Cooling Down) will help alleviate some of the soreness.

Massaging the sore muscles may also help relieve the pain but you should first consult with a physiotherapist or other professional.

Exercising above a certain threshold can cause a decreased

flow of blood to the active muscles. This can cause pain result-ing in muscle spasms. The reflex contraction causes further decreases in blood flow, which causes more reflex contractions, and so on, causing the muscle to spasm by repeatedly con-tracting. One common example of this is a painful muscle cramp. Immediate static stretching of the cramped muscle can be helpful in relieving this type of pain. However, it can sometimes make things worse by activating the stretch reflex which may cause further muscle contractions. Massaging the cramped muscle may prove more useful than stretching in relieving this type of pain.

STRETCHING WITH PAIN

If you are already experiencing some type of pain or discomfort before you begin stretching, then it is very important that you determine the cause of your pain. Once you have determined the cause of the pain, you are in a better position to decide whether or not you should attempt to stretch the affected area.

Some degree of soreness is often experienced by those who have not previously exercised or stretched – this is one penalty for having been inactive. On the other hand, well-trained ath-letes who work out at higher-than-usual levels of difficulty can also become sore. If you feel or hear something popping or tearing you should immediately stop exercising and seek pro-fessional advice. As a general rule, remember the acronym RICE when treating an injured body part:

■ Rest
■ Ice
■ Compression
■ Elevation

This will help to reduce the pain and swelling. After this seek appropriate professional advice.

STRETCHES

Choose one stretch from each category, and use the alternatives for variation.

1. BACK

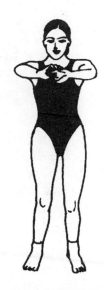

Upper Back

Stand with feet hip-width apart, knees slightly bent. Extend your arms out in front level with shoulders hands clasped and palms facing outwards (do not interlock fingers). Push forward with hands and hold.

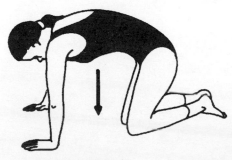

Cat Stretch

Kneel on all fours with knees apart for balance and hands shoulder-width apart. Round your back like a cat and hold. Slowly release and arch your back, pushing your stomach down towards the floor and hold.

2. SIDES
(external obliques)

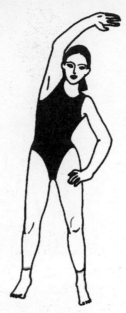

Lateral stretch

Stand with feet shoulder-width apart, knees slightly bent, toes pointing forward. Place left hand on thigh and reach up with your right arm. Lean over to the left and hold. Do not lean forwards or backwards or lock the knees. Swap arms and repeat on other side.

3. SHOULDER

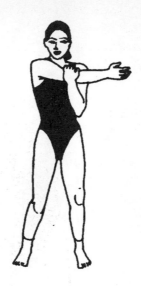

Shoulder Stretch

Stand with feet shoulder-width apart, knees slightly bent. Bring elbow of right arm across the chest and bring left arm up, bent, to hold right elbow against your chest. Pull left forearm towards body pressing on right elbow and hold. Swap arms and repeat.

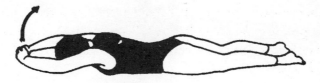

Lying Shoulder Stretch

Lie face down. Stretch arms out in front with fingers laced together palms facing out. Lift arms off floor. Hold and slowly return.

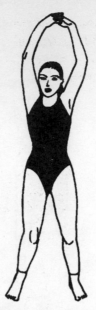

Alternative Shoulder Stretch
Extend arms straight above head with hands together. Breathe
in, stretch arms upwards and backwards and hold.

4. TRICEPS

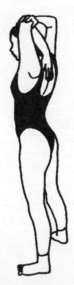

Triceps Stretch
Stand with feet hip-width apart. Place palm of right hand flat

between shoulder blades, elbow pointing upwards and bring left arm over your head to place end on the right elbow. Push down and hold. Do not push too far. Keep shoulders pulled back. Swap arms and repeat.

5. CHEST

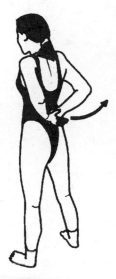

Chest

Stand with feet hip-width apart, knees slightly bent and hands clasped together behind back (do not interlock fingers) Raise your hands as high as you can behind and hold.

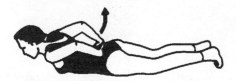

Lying Chest

Lie face down and interlace fingers behind your back. Lift arms until you feel slight discomfort. Hold.

6. BUTTOCKS

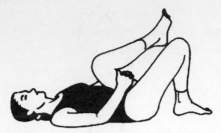

Lie on your back, keeping head on the floor and lower back flat. Pull right knee towards the chest with your hands until you feel slight discomfort in buttocks and back of leg. Hold. Slowly return leg to floor and repeat with other leg.

7. GROIN (adductors)

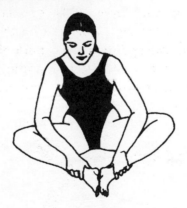

Sitting Groin

Sit with the soles of your feet together, hands and elbows resting on the inside of the knees. Look at a point 5ft in front of body and lean forward bending from hips and using your elbows to push your knees down towards the floor. Slowly return to the starting position.

8.HIP

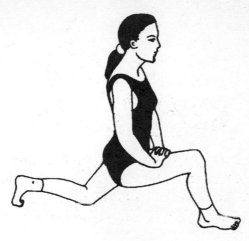

Hip Stretch

Move right leg forward, until the knee is directly above the ankle. The knee of left leg should rest on the floor. Keeping both knees in the same position, move front of right hip down until you feel it. Hold, slowly return to starting position. Swap legs and repeat. Make sure the knee of the front leg is not in front of the ankle.

9. THIGHS
(quadriceps and abductors)

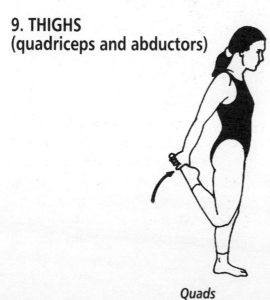

Quads

Stand, holding wall for support if necessary. Pull right ankle with right hand up towards backside. Hold and repeat with other leg.

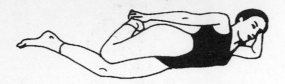

Lying Quads Stretch

Lie on left side, resting head in palm of right hand. Gently pull ankle of right leg up towards right hip. Hold. Turn on other side and repeat.

10. CALVES

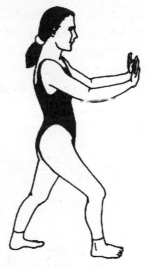

Calf Stretch

Stand short distance from wall, supporting body with arms. Front leg bent, back leg straight. Keeping back straight move hip forward until you feel calf. Make sure that back and front foot are pointing forward in same direction. To increase calf stretch put weight on outside of back foot.

11. HAMSTRINGS

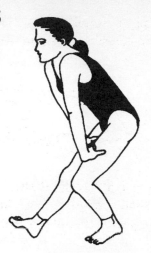

Standing Hamstrings

Stand up, bend left leg and push out right heel straight in front of you. Place hands on bent leg above the knee. Bend until you feel it in the hamstrings. Release slowly and repeat on other leg (if necessary the right foot can be placed on a step).

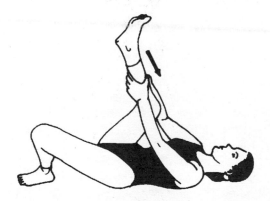

Lying Hamstrings

Lie on your back with head resting on the floor with one knee bent and foot flat on the floor. Bend the other knee in towards your chest and take the calf with both hands. Slowly pull the lower part of your leg towards you trying to straighten it as much as possible. Hold. Slowly release leg, place foot flat on floor and repeat with other leg.

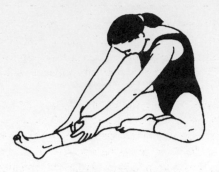

Sitting Hamstrings

Sit upright, extend right leg, place left sole against extended thigh. Holding right leg at the ankle, bend forward from the hips until you feel slight discomfort in the back of the thigh. Return slowly to starting position and repeat for other leg.

RUNNERS' STRETCHES

You can find seven other stretches that are recommended for runners in the next chapter.

JEREMY'S TRAINING TIP
HOW TO COPE WITH INJURY

The frustrating side of an injury is wondering when it is going to end and you can get back to training. My groin injury was in a deep-rooted ligament that was moving in a shearing action up and down as I was running and causing havoc to all the muscle attachments all over the place. I needed an operation to tighten up the muscle groups on the left side of the groin to give it more stability. And rest. Rest was the best cure for me. I took time out, nearly six months with no training, no playing. My family loved it but I found it very frustrating. However, I realized that this injury could mean the end of my career so I had to be patient. It is always better to rest rather than risk making it worse by being overactive too soon.

After all that time off, the motivation to get back was easy. Someone was playing in my place both for Bath and for England so I had to go out and prove a point. To cope with that feeling I told myself that if I had been fit I would have been playing for Bath and England.

To start with I set small goals like being fit for the Five Nations tournament but when I didn't achieve that it was certainly a mental and physical set back. I'm a fairly laid-back individual and I thought I dealt with the injury pretty well, but all around the England games I was very edgy and not nearly as good at coping with it as I thought. It is important to set goals that are attainable.

When I started training, it was like starting all over again. I could hardly believe I was back running and training, so in the back of my mind I was expecting my groin to go again. The longer it didn't the more I forgot about it. There were some clunks and clicks which worried me and took about six months to go. You have to learn to listen to your body and trust it.

QUESTIONS

1. Vigorous exercise increases the blood flow through muscles by a factor of 5, 8 or 10?

2. In an emergency which blood group can be transfused into anybody?

3. How many pints of blood are there in an 11 stone adult male, 7, 10 or 12?

4. Does regular exercise increase or decrease resting blood pressure?

5. It is well known that athletes should eat a lot of carbohydrates – but what percentage of their diet should be carbohydrates – is it not more than 65%, 75%, or 85%?

6. If you want to up your carbohydrate intake, Is it better to eat peanuts or pasta?

7. What percentage of British people are overweight? Is it 10%, 25% or 40%?

8. Compared to 1980 is this figure higher or lower?

9. In one level teaspoon of white sugar are there 10, 16 or 25 calories?

10. Has brown or white sugar got the most calories or are they the same?

11. The recommended maximum number of units of alcohol that a woman should drink each week is 12, 14 or 21?

12. On average, would a unit of alcohol stay in your bloodstream for 30 or 60 minutes?

13. The UK has one of the highest levels of sugar consumption in the world. How many lbs per week does the average British individual consume, 2, 4 or 6 lbs?

14. Does semi-skimmed milk contain more, less or the same amount of protein as full cream milk?

(Answers at the end of the book)

CHAPTER 4

BODY JOG : A GENTLE INTRODUCTION TO THE EXERCISE PROGRAMME

Welcome to the world of exercise where physical fitness will surely follow if you stick at it. But take it slowly. The first two weeks of our programme should be about getting used to the regularity of exercise itself. Before starting, you must say to yourself, 'I need to set aside 20–45 minutes of my life, three times a week, just to get myself moving, to get my heart and lungs going, to prepare myself for what lies ahead.'

You cannot do a hard workout if you are not fit, you are not fit if you can't get from A–B without gasping for breath. If your heart and lungs tire quickly, you are not fit. By doing some introductory heart and lung exercises for two weeks you get the blood flowing in and out of the muscles you are going to use. It is incredibly important to do proper stretching – especially if you haven't exercised those muscles for a long time. After a long absence any continuous exercise will give you stresses and strains, and muscle fatigue in places your body isn't used to. So get into the habit of warming up and stretching (for further details read the preceding chapter). If that is followed by continuous aerobic exercise, the body will get used to working for longer periods. At this stage the intensity of exercise is not as important as the length of time spent getting the body used to it.

Remember the fable of the hare and the tortoise – its moral is that jogging slow and steady, not sprinting fast and furious, wins races. That is certainly a good philosophy to adopt in training. You have made a commitment to start a training schedule that will last at least six months – and hopefully the rest of your life – so do not be in too much of hurry. Set realistic goals and you will achieve them. Your long-term goal may be to win Body Heat, and that's great and good luck, but pause and ask yourself first does it matter whether you win it next year or the year after.

The training schedules we have suggested are a guideline, based on years of practical experience, but everybody is different. If you find yourself bounding ahead then move forward in the programme. Likewise, if you realize that after two weeks of brisk walking and light jogs you are not ready to go to the gym yet, keep on exercising until you *are* ready.

For this introductory period we advise not going into the gym. Psychologically, it is better to go there when you are ready and not under any daunting external or peer group pressures. Men, in particular, have a habit of going into a gym and immediately trying to lift the heaviest weights available. Often, this results in torn muscles and serious stiffness, and is counter-productive, mentally and physically – not to say potentially dangerous.

When you start exercising for the first time after a long break you do not have to start off running. If Linford Christie has been injured he does not try to break his personal best the first time he pulls on spikes. In the weeks after the London Marathon the parks of the capital are always packed full of first-time joggers, inspired by what they saw on TV, but literally dying on their feet because their heart rate has gone through the roof. Pumping at over 85% of MHR they have gone anaerobic, their body is not used to this and they have become exhausted. Once that happens the length of time for which they can exercise is cut down.

A brisk walk is fine. Do not meander but aim to move at a steady 4 mph. To begin with it is the length of time you exercise that is important. You cannot win a marathon by training doing five 200-metre sprints a week. To begin with, it is knowing that you can actually cover the distances or exercise for 20–25 minutes that is important.

CLOTHING

All exercise clothing should be loose-fitting to permit freedom of movement, and should make the wearer feel comfortable and self-assured. As a general rule, you should wear lighter-weight clothes than temperatures might indicate. Exercise generates great amounts of body heat. Light-coloured clothing that reflects the sun's rays is cooler in the summer, and dark clothes are warmer in winter.

There is no need to behave like a lottery winner when you start exercising and go and buy up the latest fashions in leotards and skin tight Lycra shorts. Gym regulars get a great deal of amusement from watching beginners clad in brand-new expensive kit and have been known to take bets on how many times they will come back. Everyone has old t-shirts and shorts in their wardrobe, so use those until you feel you want to reward some hard work with a new exercise outfit. Exercise clothes don't have to be new but try to make them clean and sweet-smelling. If you don't already have some, buy two or three pairs of exercise socks.

When the weather is very cold, it's better to wear several layers of light-weight clothing than one or two heavy layers. The extra layers help trap heat, and it's easy to shed one of them if you become too warm. In cold weather, and in hot, sunny weather, it's a good idea to wear something on your head. Wooly hats are recommended for winter wear, and some form of tennis or sailor's hat that provides shade and can be soaked in water is good for summer. Never wear rubberized or plastic clothing. Such garments interfere with the evaporation of perspiration and can cause body temperature to rise to dangerous levels.

The most important item of equipment are your shoes. It it is easy to stint on them but don't. Cheap, poorly constructed shoes can cause injury. For running, make sure you have a pair of sturdy, properly-fitting running shoes. Training shoes with heavy, cushioned soles and arch supports are preferable to flimsy sneakers and light racing shoes. However, you should not carry out any form of circuit training or court sports (squash, badminton, tennis) in running shoes. Most running shoes provide good cushioning on the sole but not enough support in the upper if you are practising quick turns.

To begin with, we would advise investing in a good quality pair of cross trainers (look at all the best known brands like Nike, Reebok, Adidas and Asics first, they may be more expensive but they will prove worth it) which should cost around £50-£60. Make sure they are comfortable and that you can run in them without any problems. As the programme increases in intensity and your mileage clocks up, you should consider getting a pair of running shoes and keeping the cross trainers for gym work.

There is more detailed information and advice on clothes and shoes in the chapter on Running (page 122).

WEEK ONE

Three exercise sessions, each of 30–45 minutes duration. Do not exercise on consecutive days, let the muscles recover.

First, set a realistic goal, one that you can achieve. For example: 'At the end of these two weeks I want to be able to jog two miles without stopping or even slowing down for a walk'.

FIRST SESSION

Start with a 10–12 minute warm-up and stretch (see Runners' Stretches at the end of this chapter). If you have skipped the chapter on warm up and stretching please read it as it may help explain the importance of this activity to your total physical well-being. Make sure the muscles are ready and prepared for exercise. Now go for a brisk 15-minute walk. This is something your body is not used to, but the whole purpose of a fitness regime is to put your body through a resistance it is not used to. That way it improves.

Make sure you stretch at the end of each session. Some experts think it is more important to stretch at the end of a session than at the beginning. It is certainly equally important because during exercise the lactic acid builds up in the muscles and you need to be able to flush the toxins in the blood out by cooling down. A good stretch returns the muscles to their normal length.

SECOND SESSION

Do the warm-up and stretch but make the walk 20 minutes. This time choose more undulating terrain, maybe go off the path, up a small hill – anything for variation. Slow your pace over the last two or three minutes and don't forget those stretches!

THIRD SESSION

Warm up and stretch as usual (perhaps it is becoming second nature already). This time try to break into a light jog. Start with five minutes brisk walking, 5–10 minutes light jog, a further five minutes brisk walking to cool down. Stretch.

WEEK TWO

Three exercise sessions, each of 30–45 minutes duration. Do not exercise on consecutive days, let the muscles recover.
You can cut down the warm-up a bit by a couple of minutes to 8–10 minutes and concentrate on the stretching. At this stage flexibility is incredibly important and stretching will help lengthen the hamstrings and the quads because after years of relative inactivity both will be quite tight. You will also find that by the end of the week your overall flexibility will have improved enormously. After two weeks of regular stretching people who have not touched their toes in years can often manage it. Make sure the body is firing on all cylinders. Throughout the jogs this week try to keep your heart rate at the lower end of the 60–85% of MHR scale. If you are pushing the body too hard it will fatigue much faster.

FIRST SESSION

Warm up and stretch. Aim to do a 20-minute walk, jog, walk. If you feel confident, your legs are moving easily then break into the jog after 2–3 minutes not five, but if you feel shattered in the middle of the jog, slow down to a brisk walk again. Try not to stop completely as that will cause the build up of lactic acid and make it much harder to get going again. Finish the session by walking the last 2–3 minutes. Stretch after finishing.

SECOND SESSION

Warm up and stretch. Follow the same principle as the first day but try to cut the 2–3 minutes walking at the beginning and end to 1–2 minutes, or keep the longer walking period but keep jogging in the middle without having to slow down to recover. Try to jog without slowing to a walk for 12 minutes. Stretch after finishing.

THIRD SESSION

Warm up and stretch. Your aim is to jog for all 20 minutes. Do concentrate on a good strong warm up and stretch so that the muscles are warmed and pumped full of oxygen. Don't push it, just start jogging gently, after 2–3 minutes pick up the pace a little and try and hold that pace for the next 15 minutes, then gradually ease the throttle down and finish the session on a light jog. Do not forget to stretch after finishing.

Well done, you have just jogged your 2 miles. (It's easy to calculate, slow walk = 3 mph, brisk walk = 4 mph, light jog = 6 mph – or 1 mile every 10 mins.)

RUNNERS' STRETCHES

The Body Heat exercise programme starts gradually but, as running is an integral part of the competition, stretching must become a part of your daily routine. Runners, for some reason, have a reputation for hating doing stretches. They are also the first to complain once injured. Get into good habits early.

One word of advice – if you are an early bird who likes jogging before breakfast, stretching early in the morning can be difficult before you have loosened up. It is also hard to stretch before your muscles have warmed up. Be very gentle when stretching prior to a run. You might find it helpful to stretch about ½ to ¾ of a mile into your run. The muscles will have warmed up and be better prepared to be stretched.

Here are seven simple stretches that promise not to take up too much time. They work just as well when you're covering 10 miles as 1 mile so they will stand you in good stead later in the programme.

WALL PUSH-UP

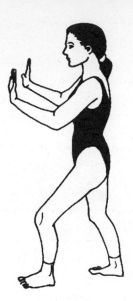

Stand with the rear foot approximately 2–3 feet from the wall. The rear leg should be straight, the front leg is bent and your hands touch the wall. Feet point straight ahead, heels are on the ground. Hold for 10 seconds, switch legs, repeat 5–10 times.

HAMSTRING STRETCH

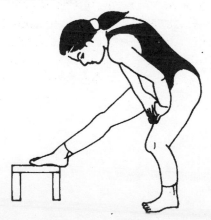

Straighten one leg, place it, with the knee locked, on a foot stool, bench or stair. Bend your body and bring your head towards the leg. Hold this position for 10 seconds. Switch sides, repeat 5–10 times.

KNEE CLASP

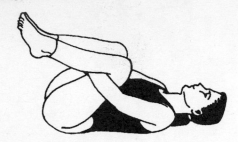

Lie on a firm surface. A carpeted floor or grass is best. Bring both knees to your chest. Hold for 10 seconds. Repeat 5 times. This stretches the hamstrings and lower back.

CHEST PUSH-UP

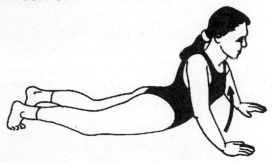

Lie on the floor with your abdomen pressed flat on to the floor. Place your hands flat on the floor, beneath your shoulders. Push your chest up with your arms and hold for 10 seconds. Repeat 5 times.

BACKWARD STRETCH

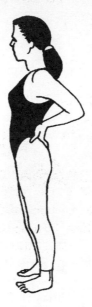

While standing straight, place the palms of your hands against the small of your back. Tighten your buttocks and bend backwards. Hold for 10 seconds, relax, repeat 5 times.

STRAIGHT LEG LIFTS

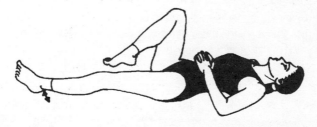

This is performed to strengthen the quadriceps. Lying on the floor, flex one knee to approximately a right angle. Lift the other leg rapidly to between 30 and 60 degrees. Lower and repeat 5–10 times. Switch legs, repeat 5 times and work up to 10 sets of 10 repetitions.

BENT LEG SIT-UP

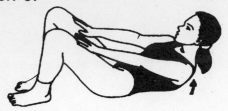

This strengthens the abdominals. The sit-up should be a gradual one rather than a rapid thrust forward. It should feel as if you are moving forward one vertebrae at a time. Lie on the floor with your knees bent. Move torso forward to a position 30 degrees from the floor. Lie back and then repeat 15–20 times.

JEREMY'S TRAINING TIP
DISCIPLINE

The hardest thing for me is to find the discipline to go out and train, even though I know success is 95% training, 5% participation. The most important thing for me is to discipline myself to train harder, to add more quality of training and to improve my skills and fitness all the time. I never used to be a hard trainer, but now I realize that to stay at the top you have to do all the hard work six days a week. At times it's boring, it gets you down on the miserable, wet, windy, cold nights you are out with your colleagues and you sometimes think 'Is it worth it?' But when you win you know it has all been worthwhile.

QUESTIONS

1. One extra average-sized slice of bread and butter a day will result in a weight gain in one year of 10, 15 or 20lbs?

2. How many hours playing squash are required to lose 1lb of fat, 5 or 7?

3. Is the average resting heart rate for a healthy adult in beats per minute, 60, 70 or 80?

4. The aorta is the largest artery in the body. Does it carry blood towards or away from the heart?

5. Vitamin C is recommended for general health. Is the recommended daily intake 40, 80 or 100mg?

6. To help preserve the Vitamin C in a baked potato is it better to bake it in a conventional or microwave oven?

7. If you stood still and did not eat how long would it be before you lost 1lb of fat – 24, 56 or 60 hours?

8. Where are your hamstrings?

9. How many pints of water are there in a healthy young man weighing 11 stone – 35, 55 or 75 pints?

10. Which organ is responsible for fluid balance?

11. How many vertebrae make up the spine, 23, 28 or 33?

12. Where is the smallest bone in the human body?

(Answers at the end of the book)

CHAPTER 5

WELCOME TO THE GYM

After your gentle two-week introduction, you are now ready to enter the gym. A gym can be a frightening place at first sight, the clatter and crash as weights meet too hard and too fast, the grunts and groans of men and women pushing themselves to the limit, the smell of both fresh and stale sweat. The sight of women in tight Lycra outfits with perfectly toned legs and bottoms, guys with bulging muscles in places you didn't know there were muscles, can all contribute to a terrible feeling of personal inadequacy. Forget that. Deep inside you know that the majority of these people were once in the same physical condition as you are now and plenty of them were far worse. So don't be overawed by the achievements of others. Given time and commitment to the cause you can surpass both them and your wildest expectations.

Many people coming into gyms get discouraged too quickly. If their goal is to lose two stone and it doesn't disappear in the first two weeks they give up. You have to be realistic in your goals, to appreciate how much it takes to actually lose a pound of fat. If your diet is junk food you can't expect that one exercise session will strip away a pound of fat (see the chapter on Body Food for a more detailed explanation of how a properly balanced diet will increase your fitness and help you lose weight). There are 3,500 calories in a pound of body fat so to lose half a stone you must drop 25,000 calories and you can't do that overnight. Starving yourself for a week would be effective but probably terminal and, if you survived, you certainly wouldn't be in shape to bench press a gerbil.

WHAT SHOULD I LOOK FOR IN A GYM?

You should find a place that can offer a constructive pro-gramme for you as an individual, not a general programme. The instructors should be friendly and helpful and there should be a good range of equipment, all of which is functioning. If you go into a gym and half the machines are out of order it will give you a pretty good idea of what sort of person looks after the place. If they don't care about their machines, are they going to care about you and your requirements?

As a joining package you should expect a full fitness test to look at your general state of fitness and heath and which will help work out your areas of improvement.

FULL FITNESS TEST

Any good gym will offer a fitness test which should comprise all or most of these elements. Obviously equipment used may vary from place to place.

1. BLOOD PRESSURE TEST

This is similar to that administered by a doctor or nurse. In a the average healthy adult this should read between 120/70 and 150/80.

2. BODY FAT PERCENTAGE

Measuring your percentage of body fat will usually be done by either skin callipers or a new machine, the body stat machine, which measures by bio-electrical impedance sending a little electrical current up your bloodstream. Andrew Nash has found in his experience there is a quite a lot of difference between the two methods. 'Callipers are better with people of a leaner build with less body fat to begin with. People with quite a lot – like your average beginner – possibly don't know whether it is fat or muscle. An overweight person can be very intimidated going into a gym and having people they hardly know pinching their fat. You do four areas, front of arm, back of arm, side of the waist and at the back (subscapular). It is prone to human error as the following week someone might measure a centimetre up or down which can give a very different result.'

Bio-electrical impedance is a computerized system that sends a tiny electrical current through the body via an electrode attached to the wrists and ankles. The amount of water in the body affects the flow of the current. Because water is found only in fat-free tissue the current flow gets translated into body fat percentage. However, various factors can cause inaccurate readings such as being dehydrated – so don't bother to get measured after an exercise session or if you have consumed any alcohol in that day. Other factors that can affect the accuracy of the readings are if a woman is suffering from pre-menstrual bloat, if you have recently eaten a large meal or if your muscles are carbo-loaded (water gets stored along with the glycogen). Another problem is that the calculations are based upon the assumption that the average person comprises 73% water. Younger people can be as high as 77%, older as low as 71%.

The point about body fat measurements is that they are all relative. What you should do is view them not as definitive statements of fact but as a measurement against itself. Make sure that the next time you are measured it is done by the same person, using the same method. That way it will reflect the changes in your body as you lose fat, gain muscle, tone up and slim down. The standard error is plus or minus 3% and there could be another 3% biological error due to individual variations. In other words being measured at 18% body fat is at best only a guideline.

3. ABDOMINAL TEST

This checks the endurance within the stomach. The instructor will see how many full range sit ups you can do. However, this is not to be undertaken if you have a bad back. If you have a history of back problems or any other long-standing muscular injury, make sure to tell the instructor.

4. FLEXIBILITY TEST

The Sit and Reach test is probably the simplest and most effective means of measuring flexibility. You sit down barefoot and reach forward pushing your fingers beyond your toes if possible. The extent of your reach can be measured on a board that measures your hip flexion in centimetres and the flexibility in your hamstrings and lower back. The average 30-year-old male will have a hip flexion of −5cm, which means they can't touch their toes. However, regular stretching sessions can improve this very quickly.

5. SPIROMETER TEST

This is a lung test to discover how much lung capacity you have, how much strength in your breath. You inhale deeply, take in as much air as you can and then exhale into a tube which measures it digitally in a flow chart. That shows your lung capacity. If you haven't got the right capacity through heredity you can't turn yourself into Mary Peters or Sebastian Coe, though regular cardiovascular workouts will enable you to increase this by 10–15%. Anything between 40–60 millilitres of air per kilogramme per minute is good.

6. SIX MINUTES ON AN EXERCISE BICYCLE

You are asked to cycle for six minutes on a cycle at a fixed resistance of wattage – for women it is between 60–120 watts, for men 150–200 watts of resistance. The aim is to work from between 40–70% of their MHR. It is not supposed to be anaerobic, but conducted at a medium level of aerobic exercise. For someone who has not exercised much they should hit a high heart rate within a couple of minutes, then it will plateau out a bit.

After this fitness test you should have a seven-page printout about yourself. A good instructor will look at the results of the fitness test, listen to what you have to say about your aims and intentions, ask whether you have any limitations, any chronic conditions or injuries and will then prescribe a programme that is within your capabilities but also in line with what you are hoping to achieve yourself. A good instructor will come across positively but be prepared to listen to what you want, to give you ideas not issue decrees, and they should say this is what you should be doing but make suggestions on how to improve.

Most gyms – as part of their public liability insurance – will insist on your being given an introduction to all the machines. In a two-hour session an instructor will give you a fitness test and then take you through what each machine does, the correct range of movement, any breathing techniques, how to set up machines for your individual height and weight. Then you should have a go on some, with the instructor making sure your back is supported in the right way, your legs are slightly bent, telling you what speed you should be doing on the aerobic machines (treadmills and cycles) and what goals you should be seeking in floors per minute on step machines.

Do not be frightened to ask instructors specific questions: How long should I spend on that machine? What intensity should I work at? What should my heart rate be? Should I be on the incline or the flat? What weights should I be using? A decent gym will have wallcharts to help explain both technique and duration. If after looking around a gym you feel that you are not getting these questions answered or that the instructor's attitude is patronizing, don't be embarrassed about looking around your area for alternatives. A gym is only as good as the instructors and the people who use it. If it has all the latest high-tech machines but instructors who can't be bothered, then forget it. Choose a fitness centre where you feel most comfortable.

You will know a great deal just from the welcome you receive when you walk into a fitness centre. People who haven't exercised regularly in the past 10–20 years will be surprised by the changes. These centres are no longer bleak, spartan places where if you don't have a cold shower after working out you aren't a real man. Many actively encourage family groups and people in the 40–70 year old age group. Fitness centres now are very concerned about keeping their clients, so it's worth while looking around, perhaps doing some pay-as-you-play sessions at different gyms until you feel happy.

Private health clubs pride themselves on better social facilities – maybe a crêche facility which is useful for mothers of pre-school children – and are good places to relax for whole families. They are also a lot more expensive. Membership fees for chic London health clubs can run over £1,200 a year.

Fitness centres are geared up for enhancing physical fitness rather than social chit chat. Prices vary but expect to pay from £30 a month for off peak use (up to 5 pm), to £45 per month for unlimited access at all times. For that you should also expect to get use of a swimming pool, sauna and jacuzzi – all good means of winding down and relaxing tired muscles after a workout.

Don't be put off by the membership fees. Look around as there are lots of local authority gyms that don't cost a fortune. Pound for pound taking exercise is one of the cheapest forms of entertainment available.

QUESTIONS

1. Which of the following is not a B vitamin – 6, 12 or 52?

2. Carrots help you see in the dark. True or false?

3. How much water does a normal person lose in a usual day? Is it about 2, 4 or 7 pints?

4. Which trace element is added to drinking water to help prevent tooth decay?

5. What percentage of calories in a portion of fried rice are provided by fat – 2%, 12%, or 22%?

6. What contains the most calories: an average portion of pilau rice or an

average-sized nan bread?

7. During exercise how many litres of oxygen do athletes consume in one minute. Is it about 5, 7 or 9 litres?

8. Which gas is found in higher concentrations in expired air than inspired air?

9. For healthy eating should fat provide not more than 26%, 35% or 40% of our total energy intake?

10. If you are looking to cut down on your fat consumption which is better greek yogurt or soured cream?

11. How many calories are there in a normal strength pint of bitter – 100, 150 or 200?

12. Which organ of the body is responsible for the breakdown of alcohol?

(Answers at the end of the book)

CHAPTER 6

GYM EXERCISE PROGRAMMES

After checking out the machines it's time to actually get going on an exercise programme that is going to keep you busy, tired and, hopefully, happy for the next six months.

In the first four weeks you must allow a minimum of an hour for each visit to the gym. If you don't have an hour then come back when you do. At this stage it is essential to do everything right, for both your mind and body are learning new things. If you rush through the exercises, perhaps not going through the full range of movement, there is only one person you are short-changing: yourself.

If time is a problem – and it's never as much of one as people claim – make sure you adapt your exercise programme properly. If you only have half an hour, don't bother to go to the gym, go for a run or do a circuit at home instead. Concentrate on the aerobic exercise, cut out all the weight machines, do your warm-up on the cycle, stretch and then do 10 minutes each on a rowing machine and the treadmill. Finish on a high, not in a rush. If there isn't enough time even for that, improvize. Go for a jog around your home or office, or perhaps try doing a circuit at home.

The exercise programme has been designed for both women and men. As it is graduated there should be no problem for either sex. If the weights are too heavy or the press ups are too hard then ask an instructor for advice. Remember this is not a battle! The programme has been divided into four sections. The first two are each of four weeks' duration, the third and the fourth of eight weeks each. The following four pages show what your schedule will be for the next six months. For convenience each of the four parts is on a separate page. It is a good idea to photocopy them so you can take the schedule to the gym with you to remind you of what exercises to do and when. After a while the exercises should become second nature.

For further information, advice on technique and other general information read the relevant chapters before starting the next phase of your programme – Aerobic Machines, Weight Machines, Floor Exercises and Turning Up the Heat, which includes both Running Training and Home Circuits. Each chapter covers the machines you will use in the order they are introduced in the programme. So, for example, before starting the gym programme read the chapter on Weight Machines and all the machines up to but not including Biceps Curls. Once you start on Weeks 5–8 read the relevant headings. The advice on Running Training and Personal Circuits is planned to come in to play after the first eight weeks, though, of course you can use it before if circumstances warrant.

EXERCISE PROGRAMME WEEKS 1–4

Commitment = Three times a week. Do not visit the gym on two consecutive days to give the muscles a chance to recover

Aerobic Exercise 24–40 minutes per session with heartbeat at 65–85% of MHR

Bike	= 6–10 mins	at 80 rpm – gears 1–5 – flat course
Row	= 6–12 mins	at 26–30 strokes per minute – low resistance
Stepper	= 4–8 mins	at steady pace
Treadmill	= 6–10 mins	at 4–7 mph (walk/light jog) – set slightly undulating course if walking

Resistance Machines: Six

Body Part	Machine	Reps	Sets	Weight
Chest	Seated Chest Press	10	2/3	Light
Shoulders	Shoulder Press	10	2/3	Light
Back	Lateral Pull Down	10	2/3	Light
Quads	Leg Extension	10	2/3	Light
Hamstrings	Leg Curls	10	2/3	Light
Lower Back	Back Extensions	12/15	2/3	Light

The weight should be set so that on the ninth and tenth repetitions it requires an increase of effort and the individual feels he/she is working.

Take 30 seconds rest between sets.

FLOOR WORK

Stomach exercises	2 sets of 20–25
Oblique Twists	2 sets of 10–15
Back Extensions	2 sets of 15–20

STRETCHES

See Chapter 3 on warming up and stretching for a list of recommended stretches – always stretch out the muscle groups you are going to be working out.

Warm Up Stretches

If you haven't time for the full warm up then stretch after the first piece of aerobic apparatus – say after your 6–10 mins on the bike. Hold each stretch for 8–15 secs.

Cool Down Stretches

After finishing your exercise session you can do a further light session on one of the aerobic machines for 4–6 mins. Then make sure you stretch out all the muscle groups you have exercised. Hold these stretches for 20–30 secs. (This will aid recovery time.)

EXERCISE PROGRAMME WEEKS 5–8

Commitment = Three times a week. Do not visit the gym on two consecutive days to give the muscles a chance to recover

Aerobic Exercise 32–48 minutes per session with heartbeat at 75–85% of MHR

Bike	= 8–12 mins	at 80–90 rpm – gears 2–6 – flat course
Row	= 6–12 mins	at 28–32 strokes per minute – medium resistance
Stepper	= 6–10 mins	at steady pace, at one-minute intervals take your hands off, then on again
Treadmill	= 8–12 mins	at 6–8 mph (light jog) – flat course

Resistance Machines: Eight

Body Part	Machine	Reps	Sets	Weight
Chest	Seated Chest Press	10	3	Medium
Shoulders	Shoulder Press	10	3	Medium
Back	Lateral Pull Down	10	3	Medium
Quads	Leg Extension	10	3	Medium
Hamstrings	Leg Curls	10	3	Medium
Lower Back	Back Extensions	15	3	Medium
ADD:				
Biceps	Bicep Curls	10	3	Medium
Triceps	Tricep Dips	10	3	Medium

(legs bent if using a chair rather than a machine)

Keep the weights set so that on the ninth and tenth repetitions it requires an increase of effort and the individual feels he/she is working. By now you should be using heavier weights, though be careful not to over do it. Increase the sets from two to three each of 10 repetitions concentrating on a full range of movement and controlled exercise form. Take 30 seconds rest between sets.

FLOOR WORK

Stomach exercises	3 sets of 20–25
Oblique Twists	3 sets of 15–20
Back Extensions	3 sets of 20–25

STRETCHES

See Chapter 3 on warming up and stretching.

Warm Up Stretches

If you haven't time for the full warm-up, then stretch after the first piece of aerobic apparatus – say after 6–10 minutes on the bike. Hold each stretch for 8–15 secs.

Cool Down Stretches

After finishing your exercise session you can do a further light session on one of the aerobic machines for 4–6 mins. Then make sure you stretch out all the muscle groups you have exercised. Hold these stretches for 20–30 secs. (This will aid recovery time.)

EXERCISE PROGRAMME WEEKS 9–16

Commitment = Four times a week. Three gym sessions – never on consecutive days; one other session, preferably running or a home circuit, make sure you have at least two days of total rest when you take no exercise at all

Aerobic Exercise 38–54 minutes per session with heartbeat at 70–85% of MHR (choose 4–5 of machines available but start with the cycle and finish with a run)

Bike	= 10–15 mins	at 80 rpm – gears 3–8 – slightly undulating course
Row	= 12–15 mins	at 30 –35 strokes per minute – medium resistance
Stepper	= 8–12 mins	at 3 minutes hands on/hands off/hands on (good for coordination and weight transfer)
Treadmill	= 1–2 miles	at 6–8 mph (run) – set slightly undulating course with 1–3% inclines
Cross-country ski machine	= 6–12 mins or 500–1300 m, Level 4–8 at steady pace	
Versa Climba	= 6–12 mins or 600–1800 ft, average 100–180 ft per minute. No resistance to setting	
Schwinn Air	= 8–12 mins or 2,000–4,000 m at 60–80 rpm	

Resistance Machines: Ten

Body Part	Machine	Reps	Sets	Weight
Chest	Seated Chest Press	10	3	Medium
Shoulders	Shoulder Press	10	3	Medium
Back	Lateral Pull Down	10	3	Medium
Quads	Leg Extension	10	3	Medium
Hamstrings	Leg Curls	10	3	Medium
Lower Back	Back Extensions	15	3	Medium
Biceps	Bicep Curls	10	3	Medium
Triceps	Tricep Dips	10	3	Medium
ADD:				
Calf muscles	Calf Raises	10	3	Lht/Med.
Legs and bum	Leg Press	10	3	Medium
	(90% maximum knee position)			

All movements should be slow and controlled, enabling more muscles to be involved with much less chance of injury.

FLOOR WORK

Stomach exercises	3 sets of 30–40
Oblique Twists	3 sets of 20–25
Back Extensions	3 sets of 20–30

STRETCHES

See the chapter on warming up and stretching.

Warm Up Stretches

If you haven't time for the full warm up then stretch after the first piece of aerobic apparatus – say after your 6–10 mins on the bike. Hold each stretch for 8–15 secs.

Cool Down Stretches

After finishing your exercise session you can do a further light session on one of the aerobic machines for 4–6 mins. Then make sure you stretch out all the muscle groups you have exercised. Hold these stretches for 20–30 seconds. (This will aid recovery time.)

INTERVAL TRAINING WEEKS 9–16

From Week 9 introduce a once weekly session of interval training on the aerobic machines. This is designed to provide both variation and a higher intensity to improve your aerobic and anaerobic capacities (for further details read the section on interval training in Chapter 11: Running). Interval training sessions are not easy to do on a treadmill as you can't push yourself to the limits because if you don't concentrate you can fall off with potentially serious consequences, so concentrate on the other machines.

To start with, keep your high intensity bursts between 15–30 secs and the recovery periods between 30–60 secs (or until you feel you have had sufficient rest to carry on). Remember, always listen to what your body is telling you.

Format: Once A week

10–12 minute warm up and stretch

Cycle: 2 mins spinning legs, gears 1–5 = 60–70 rpm
Intervals 6 × 15–30-second bursts, 80–100 rpm, gears 5–10
Recovery – 30–60 secs, gears 1–3, 60 rpm

Tips: Quick Leg Speed
Push down with one foot, pull up with the other, good hand grips, keep upper body still

or

Rowing Machine: 2 mins technique, feeling the movements
Intervals 6 × 15–30 second bursts (or 250 metres) level 10–15 at 32–40 strokes per min.
Recovery – 30–60 secs, 20 strokes per min

Tips: Explosive Power
Try to use legs, back, arms in that order during each stroke

or

Stepper: 2 mins warm up
Intervals – 6x15 secs – level 8–12 – manual setting
Keep feet flat on steps, no holding on with hands, get arms and legs pumping
Recovery – 30 secs, taking short steps with hands on, taking deep breaths

EXERCISE PROGRAMME WEEKS 17–24

Commitment = Five times a week. Three sessions in the gym, never on consecutive days; two other sessions, one running, one other personal choice; make sure you have at least one day of total rest when you take no exercise at all

Aerobic Exercise 40–60 mins per session with heartbeat at 70–85% of MHR (Choose 4–5 of machines available but start with the cycle and finish with a run)

Bike	=12–18 mins	at 80–100 rpm- gears 1–10 – Rolling Hills
Row	= 12–18 mins	at 32–38 strokes per min – medium resistance
Stepper	= 10–15 mins	at random programme (gives different resistances) – hands off
Treadmill	= 2–3 miles	at 1 mile warm up, 1 mile good pace, 1 mile warm down) – set slightly undulating course 1–3% incline
Cross-country ski machine	= 8–15 mins, 500–1600 m, Level 4–8 at Steady pace	
Versa Climba	= 8–15 mins or 600–2,000 feet, average 100–180 ft per min. No resistance to setting.	
Schwinn Air	= 8–15 mins 2,000–5,000 m at 60–80 rpm.	

Resistance Machines: Eight

Body Part	Machine	Reps	Sets	Weight
Shoulders	Shoulder Press	10	3/4	Medium
Back	Lateral Pull Down	10	3/4	Medium
Lower Back	Back Extensions	15	3/4	Medium
Biceps	Bicep Curls	10	3/4	Medium
Triceps	Tricep Dips	10	3/4	Medium
Calf muscles	Calf Raises	10	3/4	Medium
Legs and bum	Leg Press	10	3/4	Medium
ADD:				
Upper Body	Bench Press	10	3/4	Medium

FLOOR WORK

Stomach exercises	3 sets of 30–50
Oblique Twists	3 sets of 15–20
Back Extensions	3 sets of 20–30

STRETCHES

See the chapter on warming up and stretching.

Warm Up Stretches

If you haven't time for the full warm-up then stretch after the first piece of aerobic apparatus – say after 6–10 mins on the bike. Hold each stretch for 8–15 secs.

Cool Down Stretches

After finishing your exercise session you can do a further light session on one of the aerobic machines for 4–6 mins.

Then make sure you stretch out all the muscle groups you have exercised. Hold these stretches for 20–30 secs. (This will aid recovery time.)

INTERVAL TRAINING: WEEKS 17–24

This will now be of higher intensity, with more and longer training bursts and shorter recovery time.

Format: Once A week

10–12 minute warm up and stretch

Cycle: 2 mins spinning legs, gears 1–5 = 60–70 rpm
Intervals 8–12 × 20–30 second bursts, 90–110 rpm, gears 6–10
Recovery – 20–40 secs, gears 1–4, 60–70 rpm

Tips: Quick Leg Speed
Push down with one foot, pull up with the other, good hand grips, keep upper body still

or

Rowing Machine: 2 mins technique, feeling the movements
Intervals 8–12 × 20–30 sec bursts or 300m. Level 10–15 at 35–40 strokes per minute
Recovery – 20–40 secs, 25 strokes per minute

Tips: Explosive Power
Try to use legs, back, arms in that order during each stroke

or

Stepper: 2 mins warm up
Intervals – 8–12 × 20–40-sec bursts – level 9–12 – manual or hill setting
Keep feet flat on steps, no holding on with hands, get arms and legs pumping
Recovery – 15–20 secs, taking short steps with hands on taking deep breaths

or alternatively

Plyometric Sessions: Once a week maximum. Plyometrics is an extremely good method for adding explosive power to your fitness. However, if you want to incorporate plyometrics into your training routine always do it with at least one other person and make sure that the initial sessions are conducted under the supervision of someone who knows what they are doing. See Chapter 10 Turning Up The Heat (page 113) for more details on Plyometrics.

CHAPTER 7

AEROBIC MACHINES

WHY ARE WE USING SO MANY DIFFERENT MACHINES?

The reason for using different aerobic machines is simply variety. It is important to stimulate the mind as well to keep a person interested in the programme. For someone who is not used to doing long stretches on a machine it can be very off-putting to be told 'go and warm up for 20 minutes on the bike'. The repetitive nature of the exercise – and there's a lot more to see on a 20-minute bike ride outside than there is inside a gym – makes it boring. It is much better to go and spend five minutes on four different machines. This will help exercise different muscle groups but keep you mentally stimulated as well.

The driving force which sends people onto an exercise programme is usually the desire to lose weight. This does not happen overnight but it is psychologically very important as it feels as if you are doing something to speed the process along. Exercising as many different muscle groups as possible by switching from machine to machine makes you feel mentally a lot stronger.

Most gyms have weighing machines. It is important to know your weight in kilograms (even if you think in the imperial scale) as all the weight machines are in kilograms and the more advanced aerobic machines often require the exerciser to pro-gramme in their weight in kilograms when starting out. Among

67

other things, this makes it easier for the machine to calculate how many calories you burn in each session.

CYCLE MACHINE

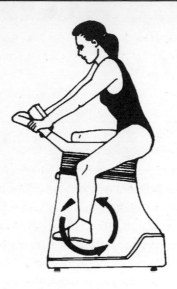

The first machine you tackle should be one where you are using your legs because they are the strongest muscles in the body. By doing a progressive non-weight-bearing exercise you are taking the pressure off other areas. It is easier to cycle than to run, climb or step, the weight transfer is different and you are using different movements. Cycling is not as energetic as rowing or running but it does the warm up very efficiently, raising your body temperature, getting the blood moving around the body, and raising your heart rate. Cycling is low impact exercise (low compression on the joints) and is recommended for any fitness level exercisers. Cycling will enhance the muscular strength and muscular endurance levels of the mid-torso muscle (abdominals and lower back) and lower body's muscle groups (hips, gluteals, quadriceps, hamstrings and calves).

Make sure that the saddle is the right height for you and that the legs aren't too straight and locked out. When the pedal is at the bottom of its revolution your leg should be slightly bent with the ball of your foot, not the arch, resting on the pedal. The ball is stronger and gives your foot more support.

STRETCH (AGAIN!)

Once you have finished the first session you are ready to stretch. We are stressing the importance of the warm up and stretch – but so should the instructor who sets your programme at the gym. If you warm up too fast your heart rate will be too high and you will not recover properly for the rest of the programme. Time and time again in gyms you see somebody rushing through their session, skipping the warm up and pounding away at the machines. Unfortunately this does more harm than good as muscles may be tight from sitting down at work and never have a chance to flex. Attacking a workout like that can lead to serious discomfort. You won't feel better at the end of it, instead you will be really tired, might get a touch of heartburn and your throat will be really dry. You will only lose body fluid which will simply be replaced the next time you eat or drink.

ROWING MACHINE

Rowing is a full body workout. You are using your arms legs and back so all your muscles need to be stretched before you do any rowing. If you have a bad back, don't use the rowing machine to begin with because the position in which you sit will make you hyperextend the lower back.

Rowing is a low to medium impact exercise (low to medium compression on the joints) and is recommended for intermediate and advanced fitness level exercisers. Rowing on the rowing machine will enhance the muscular strength and muscular endurance levels of the mid-torso muscle (abdominals and lower back) and the lower body's muscle groups (hips, gluteals, quadriceps, hamstrings and calves). Rowing also incorporates the upper back muscles (latissimus dorsi and rhomboids), shoulder muscles (deltoids and rotator cuff), triceps, biceps and forearms. The resistance level and programme selection for rowing on the rowing machine are determined by your fitness level and target heart rate zone. Increasing the speed level and/or programme level of the rowing machine will increase the difficulty level for the exerciser. Aim to stay within your target heart rate zone while rowing on the rowing machine.

When you come back on the rowing machine, make sure not to lock the legs out, the back should be kept straight and upright. Steve Redgrave – who has appeared on Body Heat twice to demonstrate the Concept rowing machine – stresses that you must get the correct movement, using the big muscle groups first. It should be legs, then back, then arm for the maximum power. It is the smaller muscle groups that give way first – the arms will get tired before the legs do. So if you are serious about competing make sure you learn how to row properly. If the technique is wrong it won't matter how strong you are.

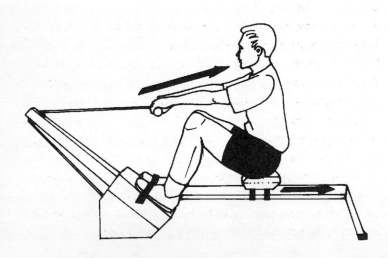

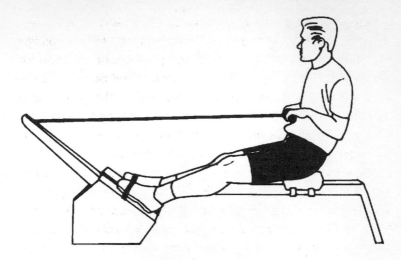

1. Begin the exercise by placing both feet on the foot boards and strap your feet into the rowing machine. The balls of the feet are to remain against the foot boards during the entire time that you are using the rowing machine.

2. Lean forward and grab hold of the handle with an overhand grip. An underhand grip may also be used, but this grip will emphasize the biceps muscles.

3. Begin the rowing motion by pushing away from the foot boards with the legs while you are simultaneously pulling the handle towards the body with the arms. Do not pull the handle first without pushing with your legs. Pulling with the upper body first may cause discomfort and/or injury to the lower back and spine.

4. After extending the legs until they are straight and the handle touches the abdominal area while pushing and pulling backwards away from the front of the rowing machine, move forward and repeat the entire movement.

5. Continue to row until you have achieved the desired time and/or heart rate level of the exercise segment.

STEP MACHINE

The object is to do a bigger range of stepping movement than in running or walking. If you watch a marathon runner, his foot hardly seems to leave the ground at all; it's as if he is sliding forward. The bigger the leg movement, the harder work it is.

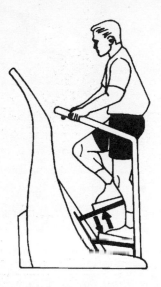

On a step you will see people doing two varieties of movement. They hold onto the side to do a small movement, travelling up and down only 6–12in. A bigger range of movement uses more muscles. It is up to the individual which they do. To begin with, a heavier person should be careful about the bigger range because you are transferring your weight from one side to the other and all your weight is going onto one leg. Sometimes people force down too hard and lock the knee out. Keep the knees soft and flexible, transfer weight evenly and think about the rhythm and the movement rather than the intensity of each explosive step.

TREADMILL

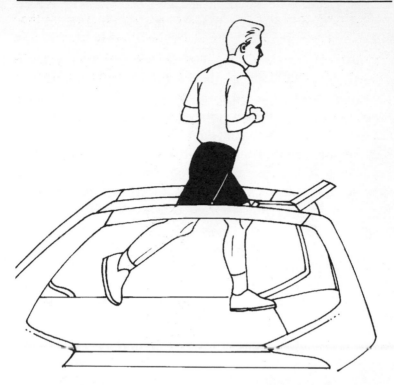

For a potential Body Heat competitor, running is the most important side of fitness. If you can't run well then you won't get on the show. Running is high impact exercise (high compression on the joints) and is recommended for intermediate and advanced fitness level exercisers. Running will enhance the muscular strength and muscular endurance levels of the mid-torso muscle (abdominals and lower back) and lower body's muscle groups (hips, gluteals, quadriceps, hamstrings and calves). Swinging the arms forward and backwards will help increase your heart rate level and tone the muscles of the upper arms and shoulders. Holding weights in the hands will increase the tone of the upper arm muscles and shoulder muscles (but do not do this early in your programme as you may never finish it!). The speeds and incline levels for running are determined by the exerciser's fitness level and target heart rate zone. Increasing the speed and/or incline level will increase the difficulty level for the exerciser. Stay within your target heart rate zone.

Walking on a treadmill is a very strange concept if you are not used to it. It's like those moving travelators at airports but more disconcerting because the treadmill has more bounce. When people stop at the end they get really dizzy and can even fall over. The secret is that if you're running at 8 mph don't just stop the machine there and then or you'll end up wobbly and disoriented or in a pile on the floor. Instead, slow the pace gradually one mile an hour from a full speed run, to a medium jog, a light jog to a brisk walk and then into a slow easy-paced stroll.

CROSS-COUNTRY SKIING MACHINE

Cross-country skiing is a low to medium impact exercise (low to medium compression on the joints) and is recommended for intermediate and advanced fitness level exercisers. Cross-country skiing on the cross-country ski machine will enhance the muscular strength and muscular endurance levels of the mid-torso muscle (abdominals and lower back) and lower body's muscle groups (hips, gluteals, quadriceps, hamstrings and calves). Cross-country skiing also incorporates the upper back muscles (latissimus dorsi and rhomboids), shoulder muscles (deltoids and rotator cuff), triceps, biceps and forearms. The resistance level and programme selection for cross-country skiing on the cross-country ski machine are determined by your fitness level and target heart rate zone. Increasing the speed level an/or programme level of the cross-country ski machine will increase the difficulty level for the exerciser. Aim to stay within your target heart rate zone while cross-country skiing.

1. Begin the exercise by placing both feet on the foot boards (skis) and insert your feet into the cross-country ski machine.

The balls of the feet should remain against the foot boards (skis) during the entire time that you are using the cross-country ski machine.

2. Lean forward and grab hold of the handles with both hands.
3. Place the hip pad against the hips and use the pad as a guide for maintaining an upright body position. Do not lean against the pad while using the cross-country ski machine.
4. Begin the cross-country skiing motion by pushing the foot boards (skis) backwards with the legs while simultaneously pulling the handle towards the sides of the body with your arms.
5. After extending the legs until they are straight and the handles cross past the plane of the body repeat the entire movement.
6. Continue to perform the skiing motion untilyou have achieved the desired time and/or heart rate level of the exercise segment.

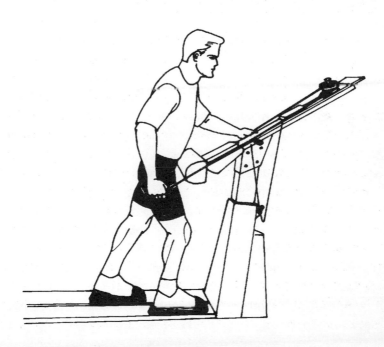

Versa Climba

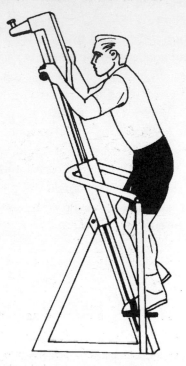

This is a climbing machine where you put your feet on the pedals, and the arms and legs move in conjunction with each other. You are on a slanted pole which you push up and down with alternate hand and leg movements. Hand grips should ideally be level with shoulders when feet are together. Start off with short steps, building up to bigger steps. Keep a tight grip on the handles pushing and pulling with each movement. It is very hard work and a movement that can be aerobic or anaerobic depending on the step distance and how fast you go. The step machine is a good introduction to the climber but be warned it is altogether much tougher. Versa climbers are not that common in British gyms and fitness centres yet, so if you see one seize an opportunity to try it out.

SCHWINN AIR

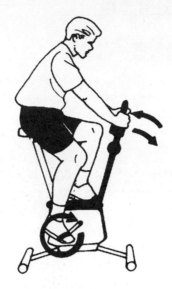

This is like an exercise cycle except it also has handles that you pull towards you and then push away. This is a good warm-up machine because you are using your arms as well. If you have a bad back, you might decide to work out using one instead of a rowing machine. As the legs are the larger muscle group use your legs predominantly, with arms pushing and pulling to help out. Concentrate on keeping a consistent leg speed.

CHAPTER 8

WEIGHT MACHINES

BASIC GUIDELINES FOR USING WEIGHT MACHINES

While machines vary according to design, age and manufacturer the basics are the same. If in doubt ask your instructors.

Do not use too much weight. This a common problem with men who often confuse lifting huge stacks with their masculinity. Make sure the weight you use is comfortable, that you can handle it. As many as one in three people suffer from bad backs, so make sure that the machines you use have a back support. A great deal of your strength comes from the midriff: if you have a strong lower back and stomach muscles everything else will follow – your glutes (bottom muscles) will be working as well. Sore joints – knees, elbows, wrists – are often caused by over-strain on that part of the body because something else is not strong enough. Bad shoes (especially high heels), bad posture, sitting incorrectly at a desk all contribute to weaknesses in the back.

Make sure you are doing the full range of movement rather than half of it. Do not sacrifice the quality of the exercise for the quantity of the weight. Do not cheat on the movement because it will lessen the effectiveness of the exercise. You are better off doing 10 reps of 20kgs than 4 reps of 50kgs – unless you are a power lifter in which case you won't do very well on Body Heat.

Most men should be able to lift 20% of their body weight

with the major muscle groups in the upper body. A woman will manage between 5 and 10%. In the legs it is higher – maybe 25–30% of body weight for men and 15–20% for women. We do not wish to sound politically incorrect or even sexist but, unless they exercise regularly, women rarely do as much with their upper body as men do. They don't tend to use their chest and arm muscles for regular day to day tasks in the same way as men do. However, women also show a very fast rate of improvement on a weight programme.

So if you are a male weighing 80kg you should be able to chest press 15–20kg easily and leg press 20–25kg. If you start with the chest press stack set at 20kg and feel a strain after 3–4 reps, then stop and drop the weight to 15kg. During the last two repetitions you should feel as if you are pushing against the resistance rather than struggling. On the next set you should find it a little harder earlier. After six or seven reps you should find yourself pushing harder.

Andrew Nash recommends that you do all your planned sets on one machine before moving on to the next. Some people do a form of circuit training where they do 30 seconds on each machine then move onto the next one and then back to the beginning again. However, for the introductory programme we recommend that you stay put. Do your first set of 10 reps, rest for 30 seconds, second set, rest, third set, then move onto the next machine. If you rest for more than 30 seconds the body has a better chance of recovering fully and you need to push each set a little harder, to put your body up against a different level of resistance.

At crowded periods in the gym there may well be other people wanting to use the machine. Polite gym etiquette is to let the other person do their set while you are resting and vice versa. Watching somebody else do better – or worse – makes the time pass quicker. As a set of 10 reps should only take 20 seconds you may also have less rest time, thus forcing those muscles to work harder.

Here is some general advice and guidelines for using the gym machines suggested in the exercise programme. However, as machines do vary from gym to gym we strongly advise that you ask the instructors to take you through the full range of movements and correct posture before starting to exercise in earnest.

Seated Chest Press

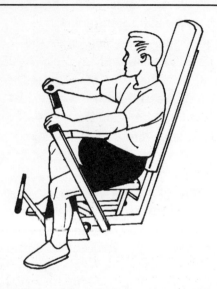

Sit down with back supported, and push the T bar forward with your legs which will bring the hand grips forward. Take hold of the outer grips making sure you have a straight line between knuckle, wrist and elbow. As you breathe out and the weights go up, push forward as you inhale. That is the recovery period and you bring the weights back slowly under control. Do not let them collapse with a crash, always keep a gap – of about an inch – between the weights you are lifting and the rest of the stack. Hold for a split second, then push forward again, not locking the arms out. It is a slow, controlled movement allowing the brain to send signals to other muscles. You do not want a jerky movement, and if you do it too quickly momentum takes over.

SHOULDER PRESS

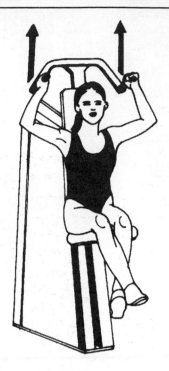

Again, it is important that the back is supported. A lot of the older machines just have a stool so that when you push up you tend to arch your back automatically. If you have something to sit back against it gives you more support. If the machine doesn't have a back rest and you either have a bad back or a tendency to arch, then use a lighter weight. Concentrate on the exercise form, making sure the stomach is tense and that you are sitting in a straight line. Push up and down in slow controlled movements, making sure the stack and the weights don't meet.

LATERAL PULL DOWN

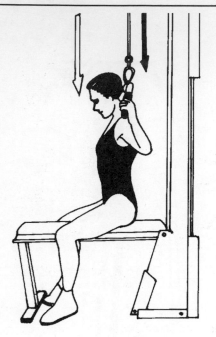

Newer machines have a bar under which you can put your knees which helps hold you down. Otherwise, if you are using a heavier weight or you are a lighter person you might find pulling the bar down that you are not in full control. You need to keep your backside firmly rooted to the seat so, when you stretch the bar up again, you are not pulling your arms out of their joints. When you pull down keep the elbows wide, bring the bar down to the front or back of the head whichever is more comfortable, hold for a split second, then push up again, a slight bend in the arms but not locked (you don't want to pull against the joint). Then pull down. You are not just using the back muscles, but the biceps at the front of the arm, the shoulders and the triceps as well. This is a good exercise for stretching out the back. If you have been sitting down all day, working on a keyboard which leaves the neck very tense, it stretches the muscles in the upper back and makes you feel you have worked the muscles all around the area.

LEG EXTENSION

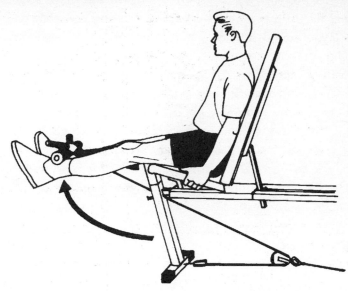

As legs are the strongest muscles in the body, beginners can start at a higher weight, maybe 25–30% of body weight for men and 15–20% for women. Sit down – make sure your back is supported – pressing the pads of the bar just above the ankle joint on the front of the leg. Then extend both legs upwards, with legs slightly bent, hold for a split second, then lower in a slow, controlled movement.

LEG CURLS

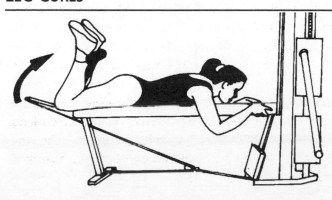

Two different types of machine work the hamstrings. Either lie on your stomach with heels underneath the roller and then bring heels up towards the backside, taking care that you do not hyperextend your back a little bit, or use the seated hamstring curl which is exactly like the Leg Extension (see above), except you put your feet over the top of the rollers and pull down towards the floor in a slow controlled movement. The hamstrings are extremely important muscles to exercise – it is easy to get strong quads (simply raising your leg does this) but the stronger the front of the leg becomes the more pressure this will exert on the hamstrings. The hamstrings are stabilizing factors in the legs and if you have weak hamstrings you will have problems – especially running.

BICEP CURLS

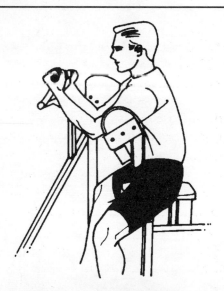

Biceps and triceps are smaller muscle groups which help out in the larger movements. Men love to have bulging biceps, and it is an obvious sign of development. Sit down and place elbows over top of the machine, making sure the elbows are in line with the pivot points. Then lift both hands together.

Alternatively, if you are using free weights (dumbbells) sit down on a hard chair or bench and do alternate arm curls, bringing the hand up towards the shoulder. Women should start on 2.5–5kg dumbbells, men 7.5–15kg.

TRICEP PUSH DOWNS

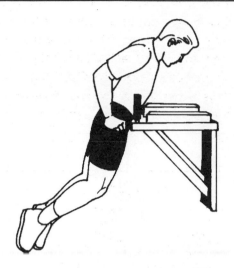

Women in particular like to tone up the triceps. If the gym has a graviton or upper body conditioner use that. This is a machine that has a pull up and a dip bar incorporated. Place your feet on a T bar and lower yourself down – the more weight you have on a machine the easier it is, it gives you a lift. As you lower yourself down, make sure you keep your elbows behind your body not out to the side.

If the gym does not have a dip machine then use a chair or bench. Sit on a chair, with hands facing forwards and resting on edge of the seat. Keeping your knees bent at 90 degrees and feet flat on floor, move knees and torso forward, so that your bottom comes off the chair supporting weight on the hands. Lower bottom towards floor, supporting weight on arms. Do not let bottom touch floor. Straighten (but do not lock) your arms to raise yourself up again. Repeat. As you get stronger straighten your legs out more so that the weight on the triceps is greater. By the end of the training programme your legs should be out completely straight.

CALF RAISES

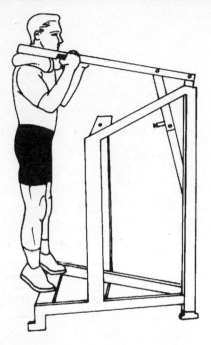

This can either be done by a free weight or on a machine. Put a bar across the shoulders and raise up and down on the toes. There are both seated and standing machines, though the standing is more common. Place shoulders onto pads, move onto step, raise on toes, slowly back onto heels. The two muscles in the calf don't require as much weight to develop as the legs. Sally Gunnell does calf raises because it adds to the explosive power of her legs. The object for her is not to get size but efficiency. This machine helps build up strength for the Body Heat endurance event – especially the machines like the rower, the step machine and the Versa climber where the calf can get tired very quickly.

LEG PRESS

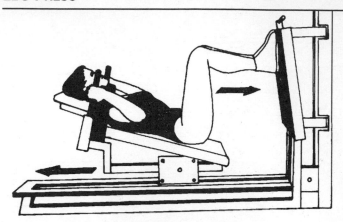

After using all the cardiovascular machines, you have exercised all the leg muscles in a full range of movement but this machine will help add muscular strength. Most gyms will either have a seated or a horizontal (lying down) leg press. On both you put your feet against a plate and push in a slow controlled movement away, then pull back towards you resisting the weights. It helps strengthen the hamstrings, the bum muscles that helps stabilize the lower back. Strong glutes are important in avoiding knee and back problems

BENCH PRESS

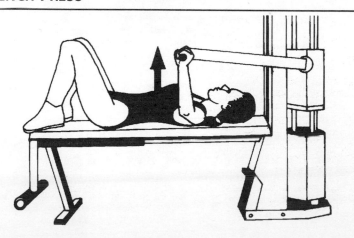

Be careful of this exercise if you have a bad back. Make sure that the back maintains its natural curve. If needs be place feet on bench, legs bent. However, if you are using free weights this exercise is not recommended as the legs form an important anchor and stability. On a machine lie on your back, feet in the air, cross your ankles, knees towards the face. Then push up in a slow controlled movement.

PEC DECK

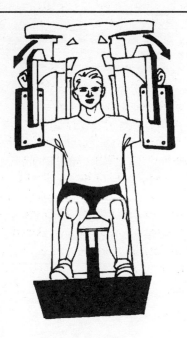

If there is a long queue to use certain machines you might wish to try alternatives. The Pec Deck is a good alternative for chest work. Ask the instructors for other options. The Pec Deck is where you squeeze your elbows together thus developing all areas of the chest. You start from the outside. As you squeeze together it works the inner chest as well. It is more of a shaping machine than a building machine. So if you are training for strength, use the chest press or bench press because you will use more muscles.

MUSCULAR STRENGTH V MUSCULAR ENDURANCE

Because the primary requirement of Body Heat is muscular endurance and stamina, we have designed this programme to reflect that. The very first event on Body Heat is the endurance test which may last only from 7–12 minutes but requires muscular endurance first, muscular strength second. At the beginning of the programme you will find that your muscles respond very well. Later on as you begin to plateau out you may need to add other types of exercise training to develop specific muscle areas.

One Body Heat test – the CYBEX machine – is purely about muscular strength. CYBEX measures both arm and leg strength, as well as explosive power. The arm test measures such a different movement that you can't really train for it other than do a series of front lateral raises with dumbbells and lateral pull-downs in front of face to chest. The leg one is easier because it is like a leg extension followed by a seated hamstring curl.

To improve muscular strength you increase the weight on the machine and lower the reps. Do four sets of 6–8 reps. If you are a man using 35kg you would go up to 45–50kg but make sure that you are still in control of the full range of movement. For full benefit you would want to do two strength sessions and one endurance session in a week. If you only do one it will give the muscles time to recover. They need time to rest but not too much.

CHAPTER 9

FLOOR EXERCISES

All men would love to have a washboard stomach – a tummy with all those muscles beautifully defined. Women would love to have firm abs too. There's only one way (unless you want to chance liposuction) to get that tone and that's lots of floor exercises aimed at firming your *abs* up.

The stomach muscles or 'abs' are designed to perform one main task, to shorten the distance between your sternum, or breastbone, and your pelvis. The only way to do this is to bend your spine in the lower back region. In short, any exercise which makes you move your sternum toward your pelvis or your pelvis toward your sternum is good. To do this safely, the lower back should be slightly rounded, not arched. In general, when exercising the abs, try to maintain the natural arch of your lower back. The lower back will round slightly as you perform the exercises. Don't fret about pressing your back into the ground. If your back aches during stomach exercises then you should consider taking a look at some alternatives.

With all sit ups you must endeavour to keep the small of your back flat on the ground/mat. If this is a problem then raise your legs and place them flat against a wall, or piece of furniture. This change of angle will keep your back flat.

You must always balance abdominal exercises with lower back exercises. If you develop your ab strength without similarly developing your spinal erectors (the muscles that straighten your lower back), you will end up with a strange and possibly damaging posture. In addition this could negate much of your machine work, as a weak back limits the amount of iron you can pump.

During floor exercises try to regulate your breathing so that you are exhaling during the exertion. For example when doing a sit up breathe in when coming down, out when coming up.

STOMACH EXERCISES

HALF SIT UPS

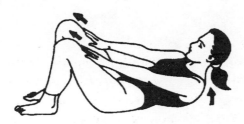

Lie on your back with knees bent and palms of hands on thighs. Sit up so hands slide up to touch knee cap. Keep your lower back on the floor. Return to start position and repeat.

SIT UPS

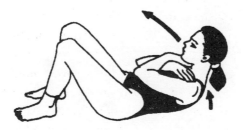

Lie on back with hands folded across your chest, knees bent, feet hip-width apart and flat on floor – if you have difficulty raising your trunk place the soles of your feet against a wall. Raise to sitting position. Lie down and repeat.

V SITS

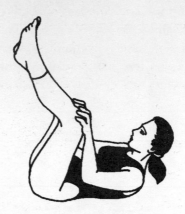

Lie on your back, bend both knees into your chest and raise both legs straight up at a 45 degree angle to the floor. Bend knees slightly. Place your hands on your knees. Raise head and shoulders off the ground, taking your hands off your knees and aiming fingers towards the feet. Return to the ground, placing your hands back on your knees and repeat. Keep your shoulders a fraction off the ground; this prevents resting and keeps the abs nice and taut.

CRUNCHES

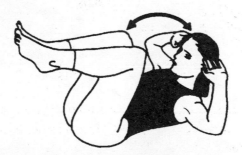

Lie on your back with knees bent, feet flat on the floor hands on temples, elbows out to the sides. Raise bent legs and torso off the ground aiming your head towards your knees. Your elbows should touch or go past your thighs. Try to do crunches as quickly and as controlled as possible.

OBLIQUES

OBLIQUES

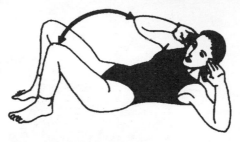

Lie on your back with hands on temples, elbows out to the sides, knees slightly bent. Sit up, bringing right elbow to touch outside of left knee. Return to starting position. Repeat with left elbow to right knee. Alternate.

ADVANCED OBLIQUES

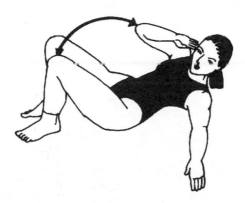

Lie on back, knees bent, feet hip-width apart and flat on floor with left hand to temple and right arm stretched out straight for balance. Raise both shoulders off the ground and twist to right as if bringing the outside of left shoulder to the right knee. Lower body down until shoulders are just off the ground and repeat. After ten raise and twists, reverse position. With right hand to temple, and left arm out straight raise shoulders and twist as if bringing right shoulder to left knee. After ten raise and twists either alternate again or stop.

BACK EXERCISES

EASY DORSAL RAISE

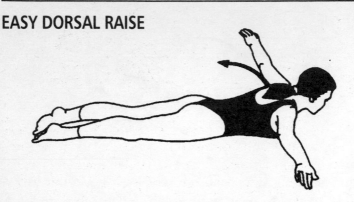

Lie flat on your stomach with your forehead on ground, arms to the side, shoulder width apart, palms flat on ground. Straighten your arms and use the strength of your back to raise trunk off the ground. Keep hips on ground. Return to start position and repeat.

DORSALS 2

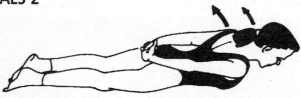

Lie on your stomach with forehead on the floor and hands interlocked behind the back, resting on the backside. Keep legs straight and lift your head, shoulders, chest as high as possible off the floor. Return to start position and repeat.

DORSALS 3

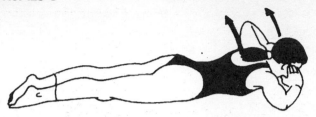

Lie on your stomach with forehead on the floor and hands stretched out in front. Bend elbows and bring hands in until fingers are touching temples. Keep legs straight and lift your head, shoulders and chest as high as possible off the floor. Return to start position and repeat.

FURTHER STOMACH EXERCISES

Recently, especially in America where having a perfect wash-board stomach is akin to having found the Holy Grail, there has been a move away from the traditional full sit up. Traditional sit ups emphasize sitting up rather than merely pulling your sternum down to meet your pelvis. The action of the psoas muscles, which run from the lower back around to the front of the thighs, is to pull the thighs closer to the torso. This is the major component in sitting up. Because of this, sit ups primarily engage the psoas, making them inefficient at exercising your abs.

They're inefficient because the psoas works best when the legs are close to straight (as they are when doing sit ups), so for most of the sit up the psoas are doing most of the work and the abs are just stabilizing. Putting the thighs at a right angle to the torso – lifting your legs up straight in the air – to begin with means that the psoas can't pull it any further, so all of the stress is placed on the abs.

Sit ups can also be a danger to your lower back. This is because to work the abs effectively you are trying to make the lower back round, but tension in the psoas encourages the lower back move into an exaggerated arch. The result is the infamous 'disc pepper grinder' effect that can give you chronic lower back pain in later life.

Bearing that in mind, we are including an alternative series of upper and lower ab exercises – don't forget to follow up with some back exercises too – which should cover the range of muscles worked by the sit ups and obliques outlined earlier. There aren't two separate muscles that you can truly isolate, so all the exercises stress the whole abdominal wall. However there are 'clusters' of muscle separated by connective tissue (these make up the 'washboard' or the 'six-pack'). You can focus on the upper clusters by moving just the torso, and the lower clusters by moving the pelvis.

Try to do sets of 15–30 reps.

You should exercise the lower abs before the upper abs and do any twisting upper ab movements before straight upper ab ones.

Pick easy exercises to start with and when you can happily do about 2 sets in a row of an exercise, try harder ones.

Only rest when you absolutely must, so take a short (10–15 sec) rest between two sets of the same exercise, but none between lower and upper abs.

Try to take about 1 second for each rep, except for ab crunches which you do slower (2 secs/rep) for a better contraction and ¼ crunches which you should do fast (2 reps/sec) because you're hardly moving.

UPPER AB EXERCISES

For the lower abs, in increasing order of difficulty you can try:

REVERSE CRUNCH

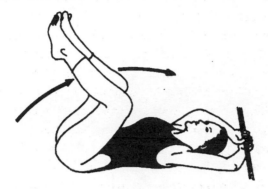

This exercise can be done on the ground or on an incline sit up board. All you need is something behind your head to hold. If you use the incline board, use it with your feet lower than your head. Lying on your back, hold a weight or a chair leg (if lying on the floor) or the foot bar (if using the sit up board). Keep the knees slightly bent. Pull your pelvis and legs up so that your knees are above your chest and then return to the first position. This exercise is very similar to a hanging knee raise, but a little less intense.

HANGING KNEE RAISES

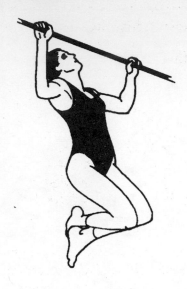

You need a pull-up bar or something you can hang from for this. Grab the bar with both hands with a grip a bit wider than your shoulders, cross your ankles and bring your knees up to your chest (or as close as you can get). Your pelvis should rock slightly forward. Pause at the top of the movement for a second and then slowly lower your knees by relaxing your abs. Don't lower your legs all the way. Repeat the movement using just your abs to raise your knees.

Make sure that you don't start swinging. You want your abs, not momentum, to do the work. It's important that you don't move your legs too far or your psoas muscle will be doing a lot of work and possibly causing as many back problems as in a sit up. Make sure your pelvis moves, your lower back stays neutral or slightly rounded, not arched, and that your abs are doing the work, not your hips.

UPPER AB EXERCISES

In increasing order of difficulty:

AB CRUNCHES

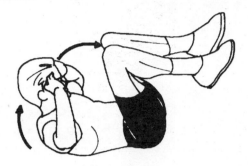

Lying on your back, put your knees up in the air so that your thighs are at a right angle to your torso, with your knees bent. If you like you can rest your feet on something, like a chair. Put your hands either behind your head or gently touching the sides of your head. Do not pull your neck forward. Now, slowly raise your shoulders off the ground and move your breastbone towards your pelvis, breathing out as you go. Although the actual movement will be very small (your upper torso should move through less than 30 degrees) you should try to go as high as possible. Only your spine should bend, your hips should not move – if the hips move, you are exercising the psoas.

Do these fairly slowly to avoid using momentum to help. You can increase the difficulty of the exercise by extending your hands out behind your head instead of keeping them at the side. Make sure you don't jerk your hands forward to help with the crunch; keep them still.

¼ CRUNCHES

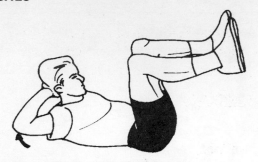

These are the same as an ab crunch except that you raise your shoulders up, instead of pulling them toward your pelvis. You can do crunches quickly, in fact it's hard to do them any other way.

CROSS-KNEE CRUNCHES

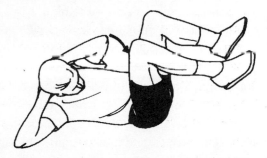

Like ab crunches, take the lying, bent-knee position, but this time crunch diagonally so that you try to touch each shoulder to the opposite hip alternately. At the top position, one shoulder and one hip should be off the ground.

BACKS

In addition to Dorsal Raises you could try some hyperextensions. We have also included the Back Lever here but do not attempt this unless you are extremely fit and in the right environment.

HYPEREXTENSIONS

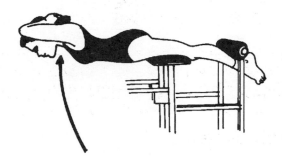

Hyperextensions are best done on a hyperextension bench, but can be done on a bed or ordinary bench with something (or somebody) holding down your ankles. Lie face down, with your hands touching the sides of your head and your body draped over the edge of the bench. Make sure your hips are supported so your pelvis can't move. Slowly raise your torso to the horizontal position, but no higher. Keep your head, shoulders and upper back arched through the whole movement. Try to do a couple of sets of around 12 reps after each ab routine or after each back routine. Don't exercise your lower back more than about three times a week.

THE BACK LEVER

(The Back Lever is an advanced exercise for people who are already well-trained. It is a gymnastic strength move, requiring a lot of upper body strength and basic gymnastic conditioning. This exercise is very tough for many people, so use caution!)

The exercise can be done on still rings, the high bar or a pull-up bar set a fair way from the ceiling. You hang upside-down with an underhand grip. If you're using a bar, the bar has to be behind you, so try hanging with the bar in front of you and walk you legs through. When you have the position, lower yourself, pivoting at your shoulders until your body is parallel to the ground (or as close as you can safely get) belly facing downwards, and hold the position for several seconds. When you can't hold it any more bring yourself back up to vertical. Take care as you have to be able to get out of any situation you get into, so don't go too low on the first try and make sure you only do it over a gym mat or with a couple of mates ready to catch you if you have to let go.

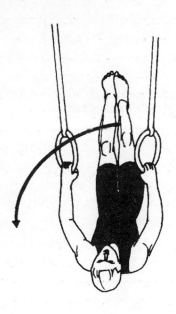

CHAPTER 10

TURNING UP THE HEAT

For the first eight weeks of the Body Heat programme, exercising three times a week will be more than enough for most people – especially those who have not taken much exercise in an age. However, there will be those who were already pretty fit or who become hooked on the whole exercise scene who will want to do more. That's brilliant, but be careful.

It is not a good idea to do weight training more than three times a week. If muscles are to gain in both strength and endurance they need a chance to rest and recuperate. Even those people who seem to be in the gym every day will be targeting different muscle groups – legs one day, upper body the next – so that each can recuperate and grow stronger.

You also need variation, because a strong body requires a strong mind. As Body Heat is primarily about endurance that is what you should be working on. So if the urge strikes to do an extra exercise session in the first eight weeks make it an aerobic one, and try to stay out of the gym. Running, cycling and going for a brisk walk in the country or even a city park are more interesting than pounding the rubber of the treadmill. There is more to see, greater variations of terrain, unexpected surprises (like things you don't want to stick to the bottom of your running shoes and ferocious jogger-eating dogs), the weather is less predictable. There is nothing like unexpected hail or a sudden thunderstorm to test the mental stamina of a runner. Do not forget to warm up, stretch and cool down properly.

A great many people play team sports – soccer, cricket, rugby, hockey, basketball, netball – or racquet sports (badminton, squash, tennis). If this was a regular part of your life before you started the Body Heat programme, don't stop it now, carry on and incorporate it. It will be interesting to see how much difference all-round fitness has made to a sports specific pastime. Once again, don't forget to warm up, stretch and cool down properly. Other people may laugh or tease you about it but if they have to limp off the pitch with a tweaked hamstring, who will have the last laugh?

Do not feel that you have to follow the dictates of the Body Heat programme as if they were holy writ. These are guidelines designed to show a gradual progression. We think it would be unwise to push on too fast with the weight training as it is important to build a strong foundation in the biggest muscle groups. If the programme is not challenging enough there is usually a simple answer – if the weights are too light just put an extra one on the stack, making sure that you can manage the full set, and employing the full range of movement. On the other hand, if you feel that you are not ready to progress – perhaps a cold or a holiday have slowed down the schedule – don't worry, progress at your own pace. If you are concerned, chat to one of the instructors.

From the beginning of week 9, the programme is adding a fourth exercise day – a gym-free exercise day designed to concentrate on improving and honing your running skills and general fitness.

As you start to get more serious in your exercise training, it starts to demand a greater commitment of your time. The serious Body Heat contenders will exercise six days a week (see Chapter 17: Winning for details of the training schedules adopted by some of the past series winners and finalists). That sort of commitment demands a very disciplined approach to training and you will quickly drop into the individual pattern that suits you.

HOME CIRCUIT TRAINING

It is important to develop a flexible attitude to training methods, so if your car breaks down and there's no other way to get to the gym you can do something else instead. Or perhaps you have gone away on holiday, there's no gym nearby and you want to keep up your strength and endurance training.

One of the best ways of doing this is a personal circuit. Circuit training is a widely used and proven method of improving muscular endurance which has been shown to produce positive changes in overall fitness, strength and speed. It can be done anywhere – a hotel room, the cabin of a cruise ship, your front room, the local park. All you need is a secure platform to step up onto, a fixed chair or bench and some flat ground.

Our recommended personal circuit (below) is tough but totally within the capabilities of anybody who has been exercising three times a week for the past 10 weeks. It is also flexible and can be adapted to suit harder physical demands. If you are continuing with the Gym Programme, then of the four days remaining, at least one should be total rest, and one or two should be running and running training. If you have taken a break from the gym programme to go on holiday this circuit can be done up to three times a week, alternating with running, but do not do it on two consecutive days to avoid the risk of muscle strain.

PERSONAL CIRCUIT

Exercises	Muscle Groups	Reps	Rest/ex
Half Sits	Abdominals, hip flexors	20 secs	10 secs
Dorsal Raise	Lower back	20 secs	10 secs
Press Ups	Arms, chest	20 secs	10 secs
Squat Thrusts	Legs	20 secs	10 secs
Sit Ups	Abdominals, hip flexors	20 secs	10 secs
Dips	Arms	20 secs	10 secs
Step Ups	Legs	20 secs	10 secs
Side Bends	Obliques, lower back	20 secs	10 secs
Crunches	Abdominals	20 secs	10 secs
Wide Arm Press Ups	Arms, chest	20 secs	10 secs
Tuck Jumps	Legs	20 secs	10 secs

3 times through each circuit
20 seconds per exercise full out
10 seconds rest between exercises
1 minute rest between circuits

VARIABLES

As with the weight machine programme, you can vary circuits to keep yourself both alert and exhausted. For example, if you simply increase the amount of time spent on each exercise, even upping it from 20–25 seconds will give you an average of three extra reps per exercise, 33 per circuit and 99 for a complete session. By the third time through you might be really shattered.

Reducing the amount of rest time between exercises would also push you harder. A real glutton might want to do shuttle sprints between exercises – that would be good practise for the bleep test. If you have the space or want to do them in the local park before starting the circuit pace out 10 metres. Do your Half Sits, then sprint 10 metres, do a quick turn sprint back and start the Dorsal Raise. First time out you'll be jogging between exercises before the circuit is complete.

You could also reduce the rest period between each of the three circuits. A minute gives the body the chance to recover quite well, 30 seconds less so. Again, you could spend the minute recovery time jogging, not lying on the ground gasping.

Alternatively you might find this too hard to begin with – especially if you start it before the third phase of the programme. If that is the case only do the first seven exercises. Always do your circuit exercises in a rotation of body, arms, legs plus at least one back exercise.

1. HALF SIT UPS

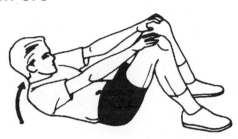

Lie on your back with knees bent, place palms of hands on thighs. Sit up so hands slide up to touch knee cap. Keep your lower back on the floor. Return to start position and repeat.

2. DORSAL RAISE

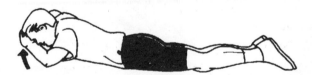

Lie on your stomach with forehead on the floor and hands stretched out in front. Bend elbows and bring hands in until fingers are touching temples. Keep legs straight and lift your head, shoulders and chest as high as possible off the floor. Return to start position and repeat.

3. PRESS UPS

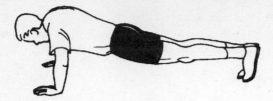

Start with hands shoulder-width apart, legs and body straight, your head in line with your body. Only the palms of the hands and the balls of the feet should remain on the floor. Keep your back straight, bend your arms and lower your chest to touch – but not rest – on the ground. Straighten the arms (but take care not to lock them) and raise the torso to return to the starting position.

4. SQUAT THRUSTS

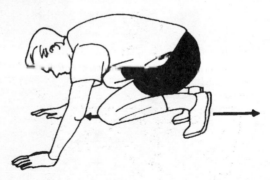

Get into press up position (arms below shoulders) with legs stretched out behind. Bring both legs forward so your knees are in line with your elbows. Thrust both legs back to the starting position. Repeat.

5. SIT UPS

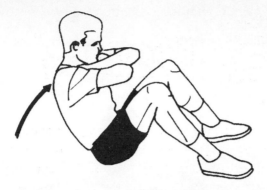

Lie on back with hands folded across your chest, knees bent, feet hip-width apart and flat on floor. Raise to sitting position. Lie down and repeat.

6. DIPS

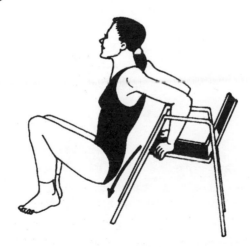

Using a sturdy hard-backed chair (or bench) that can support your weight, sit on chair with hands facing forwards resting on edge of seat. Keeping your knees bent at 90 degrees and feet flat on floor move knees and torso forward, so that your bottom comes off the chair supporting weight on hands. Lower bottom towards floor, supporting weight on arms. Do not let bottom touch floor. Straighten (but do not lock) your arms to raise yourself up again. Repeat. As you get stronger, straighten your legs out more so that the weight on the triceps is greater.

7. STEP UPS

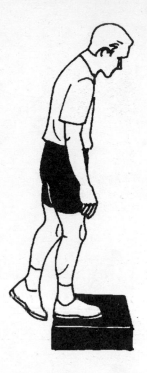

Stand in front of a box, bench, or aerobics step approximately 9in high – certainly no higher than 12in. When you step up make sure that you always straighten your leg and that the heels always make full contact with the platform. Make sure it is stable and capable of bearing your weight. Start with your right foot and step up onto the platform. Now step up with your left foot. Step back off the step with your right foot first, following with the left foot. Repeat – this time starting with your left foot first.

8. SIDE BENDS

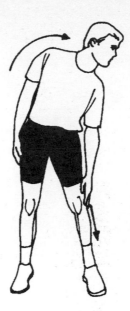

Stand with feet slightly wider than shoulder-width apart, knees relaxed and arms by your sides. Keep body upright (do not bend forwards or backwards). Lean to left side, trying to touch your knee or further down your leg. Return up through the centre and then over to the right side. Repeat, alternating from side to side but try to keep moving in a slow controlled rhythm.

9. CRUNCHES

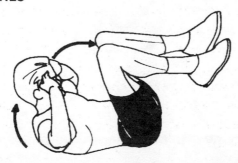

Lie on back with knees bent, feet flat on the floor, hands on temples, elbows out to the sides. Raise bent legs and torso off the ground aiming your head towards your knees. Your elbows should touch or go past your thighs. Try to do crunches as quickly as possible.

10. WIDE ARM PRESS UPS

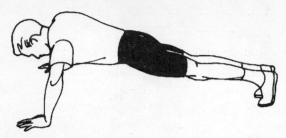

Get in the same position as the press up described above but place your arms wider apart. During the lowered position, the palms of the hands should be directly under the elbows. If you wish to make it even harder you could place your feet on a raised platform or step.

11. TUCK JUMPS

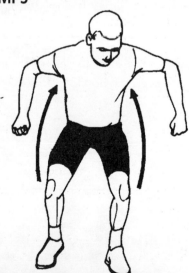

Stand with feet shoulder-width apart, your knees slightly bent. Jump as high as you can, aiming your knees up towards your chest. Do not bring your chest down to meet the knees. Make sure you bend the knees on landing – landing on straight legs can lead to injury.

Plyometrics

Plyometrics are basically a form of modified power training where only body weight is used due to the high impact nature of this technique. Plyometrics emphasizes speed of movement over anything else. The goal is to 'teach' your muscles to respond quickly and powerfully. Also, some people feel that plyometrics may improve neural pathways and improve muscle fibre recruitment over time. This makes it useful as well for athletes who don't necessarily need power but desire improved strength.

Plyometrics is one of the best ways, if not *the* best way to improve power. Power is similar to strength except you are adding the time factor. So power is the relation of strength to speed. When performing a specific resistance movement, such as jumping or bench press, the fastest person would be said to have more power in that movement. So what we are looking at is not just the contraction of the muscle, but how fast it will contract. It has been shown that a muscle will contract the fastest when it has been loaded. This is why you should be able to jump higher if you crouch down first, then immediately jump up, than if you started from the crouch.

Plyometrics relies on one of the basic facts of muscular physiology – that a pre-stretched muscle is capable of generating more force. Basically, if two conditions are achieved during the performance of plyometrics, greater force output can be realized. The two conditions are:

1. The muscle must be pre-stretched prior to the contraction.
2. This pre-stretch must occur immediately prior to the contraction.

In fact, you've already done all this. When you jump, what do you do right before leaving the ground? You bend your legs slightly so that you can jump further or higher. This preparatory movement satisfies the above two conditions. This is why high jumpers and basketball players do a quick knee flexion before jumping, so that they can go higher easier.

A good general test to see if you are ready for plyometrics is to stand and jump up as high as you can. Measure this height (chalk on your fingertips and a clean wall is a good way to measure). Then jump off an 18in box to the ground and jump as high as you can. If you can't reach as high as you could on the ground you would be better off doing more weight training and coming back in another few weeks.

Although plyometrics can be used for essentially any muscle, it is probably most frequently performed for the legs as most athletes require the majority of their strength in their legs. In all the following exercises you are using your body weight and gravity to load the muscle before contraction. The forces you generate are much larger than could be safely accomplished using conventional exercises with weights. It is true these forces only exist for a brief amount of time, but they still stress the muscle.

DEPTH JUMPS

Stand on top of a box, chair or table (make sure they are stable enough to bear your weight!) and jump to the ground. You should absorb some of the impact by bending your knees (which fulfils requirement 1) and then immediately jump as high as possible (which fulfils requirement 2). This can be performed for several repetitions. As you can imagine, the limit to plyometric exercises is really determined by one's imagination – and your fitness level.

TWO FOOT ANKLE HOP

Keeping your feet together and remaining in one place, hop up and down using only your ankles and calves. Concentrate on getting as high as you can and exploding off the ground as soon as you land.

BOX TO BOX JUMPS (high intensity)

Place two boxes that will support your weight about 3ft apart. Standing on one box step – do not jump – off to the ground and immediately jump back up to the other box. Turn around and repeat. Obviously the difficulty of this exercise is increased as the height of the boxes are increased. Once again, concentrate on getting as high as you can and exploding off the ground as soon as you land.

ZIG ZAGS

Run an elastic cord about 1ft off the ground. On one foot hop back and forth over the rope. Repeat with other foot.

SIDE TO SIDE ANKLE HOPS

Same as regular ankle hops (see above) but instead of remaining in place you jump 2–3ft side to side.

SPRINTS

Sprints are plyometrics, as the force of your body coming down loads the hamstring.

PLYOMETRIC PRESS UPS

When you first start to practise these press ups, make sure you are working on a mat to cushion yourself in case you lose control and come down to earth with a jaw-cracking thud! Usual press up position, but instead of slowly raising and lowering your body, explode the body off the floor, absorbing the impact with the hands, lowering the body slightly and then exploding again in rapid succession. The muscle is stretched before it is contracted.

PRESS UPS WITH A CLAP

Usual press up position. Lower your chest towards, but do not touch, the floor. Push up off the floor and clap hands before returning to the floor with arms bent. Raise chest back to the starting position so that your arms are straight, and repeat. Try to keep your body straight during the entire movement and make the clap loud enough to be heard.

Warning: There is a higher injury potential as this type of exercise is extremely high intensity. Generally, box height on depth jumping should be kept between 8 and 16in to minimise risk potential. Also, due to its high intensity, plyometrics should probably only be performed at limited times during the year and no more than once a week to avoid injury. Due to the high stress that will be felt on the ligaments and tendons, at least six months or more of basic weight training should be performed before incorporating plyometrics into any routine.

CHAPTER 11

RUNNING

Running is good for you.

A Body Heat champion has to have tremendous all-round fitness but the most essential skill of all has to be running. Many of the tests are running based but most of all they require endurance. Your heart and lungs need to be in good shape not only to accelerate from 0–60 in a short time but then to hold the pace at 60 for a long time. To compete successfully you need to have both aerobic endurance – an efficient means of absorbing oxygen, transporting it around the body and then using it – and muscular endurance, the capacity of your muscles to keep on going.

While the gym programme is designed to increase muscular endurance, running is among the most effective – and easiest – activities to increase aerobic endurance. Running also aids muscular endurance, but it is important to keep a variation in your running schedule as otherwise you can overwork specific muscle groups.

Most running programmes, require you to run three times a week as a minimum. This helps reinforce the habit of running, but its main purpose is to develop cardiovascular conditioning through frequent running. But more is not necessarily better. Experts in physical fitness tend to agree that running days should alternate with days of rest, since rest for the body is as much a part of developing fitness as exercise. Given that you are running in addition to the gym programme, you should not take an additional run more than once a week for the first eight weeks and not more than twice a week for the rest.

WHAT SHOULD I WEAR?

SHOES

A good pair of running shoes are worth every hard-earned penny spent. It is very easy to buy cheap sneakers and quickly incur knee injuries, Achilles tendinitis or shin splints. Go to a specialist running store and buy the best you can afford.

A good running shoe store is essential. The sales assistants at the sporting goods chain stores and general shoe stores just don't know their products or how to fit runners, despite all their advertising claims to the contrary. A real runner's store should allow you to run in the shoe on the pavement outside the store, or at least on a tread mill in the store and watch you run. The advice you get in a good store is worth the price you pay. Don't be a cheapskate and pick the brains of a good running shoe store assistant and then buy at a discount place. If you value their advice, buy a pair of shoes from the speciality running store so they will still be in business the next time you need them. Then, if you liked the pair you bought, go ahead and buy it from a discount store or mail order place in the future. Remember though, that models change, and you will want to go back to the good store every few years.

A good sales assistant will be able to tell you whether you over-pronate in a particular shoe.

Pronation and supination describe natural and normal motions of the foot during the walking or running stride. In a normal stride, the outside portion of the heel strikes the ground first. The foot pronates to absorb shock. That is, it rolls inward. At the end of the stride, the foot re-supinates – rolls outward – on push-off.

Over-pronation and over-supination are excesses of the normal motions. Over-supination is very rare. Most people who think they over-supinate probably just under-pronate. Some people who think they over-pronate may in fact pronate a normal amount, but fail to re-supinate sufficiently at the end of the stride. If that sounds complicated don't worry: over-pronation is fairly common and many shoes are designed to counteract this. But if you do have an excessive roll, either in or out, it might be necessary to see a podiatrist who will make you some orthotic insoles to put inside your shoes and help correct the imbalance.

Expect to pay from £70–£120 for a good pair of running shoes more than a good pair of cross trainers. For that money demand and expect proper service. Don't just say, 'oh that looks cool'. Look at them carefully and see whether they match your requirements. Nike, Reebok, Adidas, Puma, Asics and Brooks all make high quality trainers, but do not be fooled by the latest gimmick. A running shoe with the latest air-filled sole will still not make you a hovercraft. If you buy a car you look at the engine, with a pair of shoes look at their construction.

If you remove the insole, you can tell the type of construction. The last is the form the shoe is made on. Lasts vary from curved, to semi-curved, to straight. Straight lasts are generally the most stable shoes, while curved lasted shoes tend to be the most flexible. You just have to see what last, from what manufacturer fits your foot. Slip-lasted shoes have a sewn seam running the length of the shoe. Board lasted shoes have a cardboard board running the length of the shoe. Combination lasted shoes have cardboard in the rear half, and a seam up the front half. Slip-lasted shoes are the most flexible. Board lasted shoes are the most stable and least flexible. Combination lasted shoes attempt to compromise giving a flexible forefoot and a stable rear. Orthotics wearers should stick to board- or combination-lasted shoes. True over-supinators (these are rare) should use flexible slip lasted shoes. Another way to look at it: if you have a rigid foot (possibly high arched), favour flexible (slip-last) shoes. If you have a floppy foot (tends to have flatter feet and over-pronate), favour combination or board construction.

CLOTHES

It is possible to spend a fortune on buying all the trendiest, flashiest running gear, but whizzo stripes do not make you a jet engine. Wear whatever is most comfortable for you. Remember that as you run further, harder and faster the body gets warmed up so you do not want to be over dressed. Similarly if it is cold and you wear too little you can be uncomfortable, or worse, cause muscular strains.

In warm weather a running vest or a t-shirt over shorts is fine. Some people favour caps to keep the sun out of their eyes, with sweat bands on wrist or forehead. Always have at least two sets of running equipment as old clothes are both smelly and unhygienic the next day. Always put on a clean pair of running socks.

The rules for winter and cold weather running are different. The first rule is to dress in layers: outer layers can be added/shed easily. The second rule is to stay dry. When your clothes get wet, they get very heavy – heavy enough to degrade performance – and you get cold. The third and final rule is you must hydrate. You may not sweat as much, but you still need to take in fluids – probably more than you think.

The layer closest to the skin should be a tight, lightweight fabric that 'wicks' water away from the skin. Shirts should be long-sleeved, skintight (without chafing), and may be turtle-necked (you lose a massive amount of heat through the head and neck in cold weather). Lycra running tights work very well. The next layer should be a looser, medium-weight fabric that wicks water. A zipper at the neck is convenient for temperature control. Two layers of Lycra tights work if it's really cold. A water-proof or water-resistant shell that is breathable is useful in the coldest conditions. These are usually sold as suits, but tops are available separately at a higher cost. Gore-tex is considered by many to be the best fabric. Gore-tex is a teflon-based membrane with microscopic holes whose claim to fame is that it will let water vapour (from sweat) out, but not liquid water (rain) in. It blocks wind fairly well too. The membrane is delicate, so it always comes laminated between two layers of other material. Although effective because it is the market leader and a known brand name, it is pricey. There are less expensive alternatives.

Many people run in sweat pants, but sweats have two disadvantages: they're heavy and they get heavier when wet. Lycra is lightweight and warm, but costs more and shows off body imperfections more than sweats. There are also cold weather running tights available from specialist shops. In really cold weather pull on gloves made of cotton (wool tends to get very sweaty) or a breathable fabric. A lot of heat is lost through the scalp, so a hat is a must for most people. Cotton hats get too heavy with sweat. Balaclavas are more versatile than hats, and allow you to cover your neck/face if required.

Anybody who runs at night – in town or country – should invest in a reflective strip. Car drivers are notoriously bad at judging runners' speeds and should be given as much opportunity to miss you as possible.

WHERE SHOULD I RUN?

This is entirely up to you and your personal feelings about running on a treadmill or outside, braving the elements. There are advantages to both. It is good to run on treadmills because it takes away the pressures on your knees and ankles. Good modern machines have a bounce in them which is far better than running on concrete. On a treadmill you have a set pace for running. If you are feeling good you can speed it up, and set different inclines which mentally gives you a set focus. It can stop you working too hard, and regulates your speed. Sometimes, if you are out running by yourself, you feel you are not working hard enough and you can come back shattered. A treadmill is the best way of getting accurate speed, distance and time measurements which is very encouraging. Just set the controls, warm up, and then run your set distance. Then you can say, 'I can run 2 miles in 14 minutes, no problems'.

However to many people running inside on a treadmill can get very boring. And there is no fresh air. On a warm day what can be better than going for a run over the moors, or through a wood, or along the beach at sunset? There is plenty to see and the time passes very quickly. The important thing with running outside is to keep variety (yes, that again), to change your routes regularly, and to keep setting new time and distance targets.

And when it comes to the Body Heat Finals – which is what you're aiming at, after all – those take place outside. In the big outdoors there is always the unexpected.

WHEN SHOULD I RUN?

Is it better to run in the morning or evening? It's important to establish a routine for yourself, geared to your own disposition and living habits. Some runners prefer to run early in the morning, some even before daybreak. They seem to like the solitude available at that hour, when the streets are still empty of traffic and people. Some runners are shrewd enough to kill two birds with one stone. They get their exercise in while 'commuting' to work. People who do their running in the morning say that it sets them up for the day. They are more alert and less likely to become upset by the pressures and frustrations of their work, and at the end of the day they feel less fatigued.

Other runners wait to run after work, when they have put their jobs behind them, and headed home. A run at this time provides a nice transition for them, a time to work off some of the tensions that may have built up during the day so that they don't carry them into family life. You should end your run at least an hour before you retire, otherwise you may find it difficult to fall asleep.

As with your visits to the gym choose what time is best for you and your lifestyle. If you haven't got time to go to the gym, a hard run (including warm-up and stretch) can be completed in 35 minutes.

RUNNING TRAINING

Here are some pointers on how to maximize your running with advice on how to increase both distances and speed.

Should I Warm up, cool down and Stretch?
You need to ask?

Of course. Stretching is essential to avoid injuries. See the list of Runners Stretches on page 44.

JOGGING

Jogging – or a continuous run over a long period of time – is the perfect beginning to provide the foundation stone on which to build your future fitness. Regular running improves the cardio-respiratory system, allowing more air to reach the blood as it is pumped through the lungs. This also increases the capacity of the blood to carry oxygen to the muscles. A steady rate of exercise allows the working capacity of the heart to increase, and it becomes more efficient, leading to a subsequent drop in the pulse rate. As you get fitter you will notice that your pulse rate is lower when you are at rest or even during exercise. When you start out doing a three-mile course your heart rate will start high and then plateau off as your body gets used to the demands being placed upon it. Let us say that during the middle period your heart rate is 152 bpm. After six weeks of regular jogging you may well find that at the same point in the run it has dropped to 146 bpm.

As you continue to exercise, your cardiovascular system will open up under-developed blood vessels and develop new capillaries in the muscles which will in turn provide a better blood circulation round the body.

These physical improvements occur over time. Buying a pair of running shoes, snazzy Lycra body suits and then heading off into the sunset at full speed is more likely to cause heart failure than improved performance. Progression is the name of the game, starting with small distances and low intensity of effort.

You saw how it was possible to jog two miles, without killing yourself, after only two weeks. By following that approach it is easy to build up to a standard training run of between two and five miles.

Once you have built your running base, start on a series of runs over a measured distance and time each run. Each day try to reduce the time. Start with a circuit of between one and two miles long. As the running becomes easier, the distance should be increased while simultaneously trying to reduce the time.

Remember, keep the goals achievable. You might start with an average pace of nine minutes a mile over two miles. Six weeks later you might hope to be running four miles at an eight minutes to the mile pace. Alternatively you could start running at a steady pace for 15 minutes. As you get fitter the distance you run will increase though the time remains the same.

Variations on a Jog

Once your running base is built, to be able to compete effectively it is necessary to improve upon your overall speed, your acceleration and your general stamina. Too many joggers let themselves sink into a routine, they follow the same route day in day out, or they set the treadmill for the same speed and the same distance every trip to the gym. One-paced jogging gets pretty boring but, worse, it can lead to injuries. If you continue running the same route at the same pace you will only ever use the same muscles, and the repetition, especially if you are running on concrete or tarmac, can lead to strain or injury. It is not just your brain, but your body too that needs change and variety.

FARTLEK (varied pace running)

If you force your body into anaerobic activity (which means the body working without oxygen) – say with a sudden sprint – the subsequent oxygen debt will demand an opportunity to recover once you have slowed down to an easier paced jog.

This acts as a stimulus for the body to improve both its maximum oxygen intake and speed of recovery. Thus it improves endurance and your ability to tolerate and recover from running faster.

Fartlek – Swedish for 'speed play' – was originally developed to refresh athletes on a tightly controlled track programme. Find a varied terrain full of inclines, with different running surfaces – sand, grass, concrete, mud – along wooded paths, over sand dunes, along river banks, anything to keep you on your running toes. While fartlek should be viewed as fun, an exhilarating change that is better than a rest, it should be planned properly, matching overload situations with recovery phases.

A typical fartlek session could last 30 minutes divided as follows:

Jogging – 5 mins
Fast evenly paced run – 3 mins
Brisk walk – 2 mins
Evenly-paced running with 50–60m sprints every 200m–5 mins
Jogging   2 mins
Evenly-paced running with occasional inclusion of 4–5 fast strides, small acceleration sprints – 3 mins
Jogging with one fast uphill run (20–30m) in every min – 5 mins
Jogging and rhythmical exercise, skipping, general knee raises – 5 mins

Don't forget to stretch at the end of the session.

You can also bring fartlek techniques in to your normal run. Sprint 200m, walk the next 200 or use lampposts as markers. To push it harder decrease the jog times, so it's sprint three lamp posts, jog just one, then start again. Endurance training should involve a variety of conditions so that your body can react to change. Throw a long hill in, trying to keep the same pace going up the hill which works you harder so the heart rate goes up and down, up and down. One way to keep your heart rate up is to do more pumping with the arms like a sprinter. A distance runner hardly lifts his heels and there is no knee lift.

INTERVAL TRAINING

Interval training consists of running a specified number of distance – from 100–1000m – in a given time, with short recoveries or rest periods in between. When bouts of heavy work are interspersed with short rest periods, the total work load is much higher than it would have been over one single continuous run.

As with fartlek, make sure you have a good aerobic base when you start, and don't do too much too fast. You can tire your muscles out, and it will take a while to recover. Your goal is to exercise your fast twitch muscles, those used for speed. The process will improve both aerobic and anaerobic capabilities. Remember to warm up, cool down and stretch sufficiently before and after interval training sessions. Take at least 10 minutes of jogging to warm up and five to cool down.

The principle is simple. Let's say your goal is to run a consistent 8-minute mile over five miles. To do a mile in 8 minutes means you have to do 400m in two minutes or under. Start your intervals by doing five runs of 400m at a little under 2 minutes per rep. In between each rep you have a recovery period of 30–60 seconds depending on fitness. After five reps take a minute's rest and then continue for a total of six sets of five reps. The number of reps you will do depends on your aims but it should relate to the intensity of your training. The harder you work the fewer reps you need run.

Keep in mind that the interval part of the run is the rest part. This is where your body recovers and strengthens itself. Try to keep jogging or walking during the rest interval as some form of light exercise will help your muscles clear themselves of lactic acid and other waste products, thus producing a better and speedier recovery. Remember to keep with what you started at. If you jogged to rest in the first interval, don't walk during the next one.

Intervals should be challenging, but not defeating. If you are having problems maintaining your form during the course of the whole run, you are doing too much. You should feel good at the end of your run, not ready to drop dead. You can customise intervals to achieve different things. For example, to increase endurance, you can decrease your interval time while running the same number of reps. Or you can increase the reps and still do the same interval. You can work on speed by running faster reps.

GRID SPRINTS

Grid Sprints are anaerobic exercises which means the body is being pushed to its very limits, using a non-oxygen energy supply. Because they require intense bursts of exercise followed by sharp turns they can be a useful training tool for the dreaded 'bleep test'.

Find a flat space of ground, indoors or outdoors, that measures 20m. Mark every 5m (anything will do – a sweatshirt, a fizzy drink can, this book – it is only a mark, not something you have to avoid). Start with a 10-minute jog and stretch.

You can either do them short then long, or long then short.

Short then Long
1. Run start line to 5m mark and back.
   Run start line to 10m mark and back.
   Run start line to 15m mark and back.
   Run start line to 20m mark and back.
2. Rest for 30 secs then repeat.
3. Rest 30 secs then sprint.
   Start line to 10m mark and back.
   Start line to 20m mark and back.
4. For long ones sprint start line to 20m mark and back three times.
5. Take up to 2 mins breather then repeat up to 3 times depending on fitness level.

Long then Short
Start with the 3x20m mark sprints (4) and do the cycle in reverse.

HILL SESSION

While running up hills and inclines of varying steepness should be a regular part of your training, there might be occasions when you want an anaerobic blitz. When running up hills, try to keep the same pace all the way up to and over the brow. If you slow before the top it always seems to take much longer to make it to the top and hurts much more. The idea is to stride forward keeping good form and shape. If your head is going from side to side it means you are getting too tired. Also be careful when running down hills. It's easy to go too fast, you are using different muscles and could cause a strain

First find a hill with a clear running area up to 100m long, the gradient should be 1 in 5 or 6 – not too steep. Start with a 10-minute jog and stretch.

1. Start running at the bottom, a steady pace that increases to become progressively faster and harder by the top.
2. Slow jog down.
3. Repeat twice more without stopping.
4. Take 2 mins rest, try to keep moving either with a brisk walk or a slow jog.
5. Second set of three reps, followed by 2 mins rest.
6. Third set of three reps, followed by 2 mins rest.

(If you feel really macho, try doing the whole session without a break. Nine times up and down without a breather should sort out even the fittest).

During a recent respite from filming the 1996 series of Body Heat, Andrew Nash took both Sally Gunnell and Jeremy Guscott on a hill session (Mike Smith preferred to go swimming!).

'We chose a hill with a 10% incline, with a track of about 50m going up it', says Andrew, 'not too steep but enough to know you are going uphill. We started with a 10 minute jog to warm up, did some stretches and then went for it. Six 50m sprints, 2 mins rest, same again twice more through. The whole exercise session only took 20 mins but everybody felt they had really pushed themselves. However, a hill session like that is something to do with a group or at least one other person there. If you tackle those sessions alone you can train too hard or not hard enough and lose perspective.'

Because this is an anaerobic exercise do not do it more than twice a week.

RUNNERS TIPS

WEATHER CONDITIONS

Cold weather should not present any serious problems for you, especially if you are in reasonably good condition, and you are wearing the right clothes (see above). High wind-chill factors are the greatest threats to you in cold weather, since you can suffer frostbite if you are not adequately protected from the wind. You must remember that when you run, your own motion against the wind increases both the windchill factor and the risk of frostbite. If there is a strong, chill wind, start your session running into the wind for the logical reason that if you run downwind, start sweating and then turn around, you will freeze on the way back. At cold temperatures the amount of sweat is still great, and dangerous if you start to freeze. In really cold temperatures you want the hard part of going into the wind first so you don't get caught out longer than you can cope. When you run in cold weather, beware of ice on the road, and remember to taper off your run slowly so you will not catch a chill. Be sure all normally exposed areas of skin are covered: head, face, ears and hands. The important thing to remember is that you must dress in layers in order to create your own insulation. When you arrive home, change out of your damp, sweaty clothes right away.

When you run in hot weather you can suffer heat exhaustion.

If you start feeling dizzy and dehydrated while jogging and your pulse and breathing grow very rapid, you could very well be on your way to heat exhaustion. Stop exercising immediately. Get out of the sun, drink fluids (tepid, not cold), and rest.

Running in heat also slows down the blood circulation, placing a greater burden on your heart. And of course, you will sweat a lot more so your body loses more water that usual. To replace it, drink a full glass of water before you start and one every 15 or 20 minutes during your run. A few pinches of salt dissolved in the water will help. If your stomach is empty, omit the salt or it may cause stomach cramps. An important thing to remember about hot weather is that it takes your body about two weeks to adjust.

If you run in a strong wind, you will expend 6% more oxygen than you would under ordinary conditions. So, if you are running in a stiff breeze, slow down and you will get the same benefits as you would from a faster run. When you set out on a windy day, start with the wind in front of you at the beginning of your workout; then, at the end, when you are more tired, you will have it at your back, helping to push you along.

Rain need not be a deterrent unless you're afraid of melting, but you will need some protection. Wear waterproof outer clothes, of course, and as many layers as you need to keep warm. Don't linger in them after the run but get into dry things as soon as you get home.

High altitudes are a source of special problems. When you get to 5,000ft above sea level and beyond, it takes a lot more time for oxygen to be absorbed into your blood and travel throughout your body. So your heart has to work a lot harder at its job. Plan on taking at least four to six weeks to get adjusted to a new high altitude, and adapt your jogging routine accordingly. Most runners recommend cutting your programme by about 50% at the beginning. However after running for a while at high altitude you will find that your performance closer to sea level is much improved.

ILLNESS AND EXHAUSTION

There are certain times when you have no business running. If, for example, you have the flu, a cold, or some other ailment, don't overexert yourself and possibly harm your body by trying to run. If you feel a cold coming on, however, running may help you get rid of it. But if you decide to try this cure, follow these recommendations: dress warmly, take two aspirin in a glass of milk, and then go out for a run. Jog slowly and see how you feel. Continue jogging until your body grows warm, even hot. Then try to keep your temperature at that level.

In Britain we talk about 'hitting the wall', in America they call it 'bonking'. Lots of people talk about the phenomenon which hits some people harder than others. It happens, especially on long runs, when you literally think you've run into a wall and can go no further. It is a combination of two processes. The first is a lack of muscle glycogen. The second is low blood glucose. When muscle glycogen is low the muscle runs into a fuel crisis. It cannot burn fats at a rate high enough to sustain the muscle's maximal output. The consequence is that your muscle has to rely on burning more fats and so you have to slow down. The ghastly feeling that you experience at the same time, often characterized by nausea and disorientation, is probably a consequence of low blood sugar/glucose (hypoglycemia).

The trick then is to prevent the onset of these symptoms by ensuring that you have a high carbohydrate diet, or simply to become so well-trained that you don't have to worry. Why is low blood sugar bad?

Because your brain, eye tissue, and other organs are able to burn only glucose. That is, when the levels of glucose are low, your brain runs out of fuel, so you feel awful. Your vision might become impaired also.

A good training schedule should allow you to run over the wall or even through it. You won't feel like bonking at the end of it but, once its happened, you'll know how to deal with it in the future.

If you get a sharp muscular pain when running stop immediately and massage the aching area. If it feels better continue slowly, but if the pain comes back again stop and walk home. Apply the standard RICE technique (see page 26) and if the symptoms persist see a doctor. Listen to your body. It is the best indicator of potential problems.

CALORIE BURNING

To end this chapter on a positive note here is a chart that will show you approximately how many calories you will consume in an hour running relative to your weight and the pace you travel at

Weight (lbs)	Calories burned per hour running								
	12.00	10.43	9.41	8.46	8.02	7.26	6.54	6.26	6.02
				(Pace – minutes per mile)					
100	400	450	500	550	600	650	700	750	800
119	432	486	540	594	648	702	756	810	864
128	464	522	580	638	696	754	812	870	928
137	496	558	620	682	744	806	868	930	992
146	528	594	660	726	792	858	924	990	1056
154	560	630	700	770	840	910	980	1050	1120
163	592	666	740	814	888	962	1036	1110	1184
172	624	702	780	858	936	1014	1092	1170	1248
181	656	738	820	902	984	1066	1148	1230	1312
190	688	774	860	946	1032	1118	1204	1290	1376
199	720	810	900	990	1080	1170	1260	1350	1440
207	752	846	940	1034	1128	1222	1316	1410	1504
216	784	882	980	1078	1176	1274	1372	1470	1568
225	816	918	1020	1122	1224	1326	1428	1530	1632
234	848	954	1060	1166	1272	1378	1484	1590	1696

Note: *These figures are relative to the individual and their state of fitness and they should not be used as an absolute guide.*

CHAPTER 12

BODY FOOD 1: FUEL FOR FITNESS

Do you want to be Fat or Fit ?

For lunch before the World Cup Final in 1966, the England Team sat down to a nourishing meal of steak and chips. 'That was what we ate in those days,' comments Geoff Hurst, who scored a memorable hat-trick that day. 'Steak was supposed to be good for you, to build up your strength. All the boxers we knew would eat loads of red meat.' One of the comic book heroes of the time was Alf Tupper, the 'Tough of the Track', a working-class runner who won all his races on a diet of fish and chips.

Not any more. Today before such a big match, footballers will eat a carefully balanced meal of white meat, fish and loads of pasta. Sports nutrition is an art that can give that extra reserve of energy, convert those last grams of excess fat into energy. All professional athletes will follow a strict diet regime. Or at least they will claim to. However, like most mortals, athletes are open to temptation, to chocolate bars and pints of beer, to fast food burgers and cream buns. We are all surrounded by a torrent of – often conflicting – information about this diet and that diet. The result is that most of us know what we should eat. We just don't do it.

Most people put on weight as they get older, a few inches on the stomach for men, on the hips for women. It is a part of life which can be reversed. But it's hard work, especially if you have not taken regular exercise for a long time. And it is not just older people either. There is an increasing problem in Britain with young adults and schoolchildren who have a poor diet and take little exercise, preferring to play computer games to the rigours of football or even of croquet. A 1995 report into obesity from the Nutrition and Physical Activity Task Forces found that 57% of the male population is either overweight or obese – a frightening statistic. From 1980–93 the percentage of the adult male population that was clinically obese had risen from 6 to 13%. On current trends that will reach 18% by 2005. The percentage of overweight adult men had risen from 33% to 44%. In 1992 36% of women in the UK were found to be overweight and 12% were classified as obese.

It is time to face facts. You can only put on weight if you eat more calories than you consume in your daily activities. The only sure fire way to lose weight is to eat less and exercise more. Fat people are fat because they eat too much. Being fat is a state of mind, a psychological addiction that can be as hard to kick as heroin. As a nation we are in danger of succumbing to passive fatness. An endless litany of excuses, all of which begin: 'poor them, it's not their fault . . . they've got a slow metabolism . . . it's a medical, not a behavioural problem . . . it's their hormones . . . it's in their genes'.

That slow metabolism argument only applies to a small number of people. The problem for most of us is that we are all much less energetic than we think we are. The average woman expends only 50% more energy in a day than she would have had she stayed in bed. In our world of cars and other labour saving devices it's getting harder to stay in shape just by existing. It is an illusion that fat people are naturally indolent and less active physically. Carting that extra weight around, fat people burn up more energy than thin ones. So if fat people use more energy than thin ones how come they're fat?

They lie. Perhaps this is a sin by omission but they lie, to their partners, to researchers, but most of all they lie to themselves. 'This myth about slow metabolism has come about because overweight people always underestimate what they eat. Fat people aren't going to like this, but it's incontrovertible,' says

Dr Andrew Prentice, head of Obesity Research at the Dunn Clinical Nutrition Centre. In a 1991 report his team discovered that their subjects consistently underestimated their food consumption by an average 833 calories a day. As the recommended daily intake for men is 2,500–3,000 calories, and for women 2,200, this helps to explain away a lot of unaccounted-for fat.

Except for that tiny percentage of the population who do suffer from underactive thyroids and pituitary disturbances, the majority of obese people are obese because they eat too much. 'Acute medical conditions are very rare,' explains Dr Peter Kopelman, a senior lecturer in Medicine at the Royal London Hospital. 'The Prader-Willi syndrome, where a lesion in the brain means there is no appetite control, is only found in 1 out of 60,000 people. Similarly, while starvation diets cause the body to slow your metabolism down, if you return to a normal diet it speeds up again. Fat is a mental thing, you have to learn to control eating and motivate yourself to take more exercise.'

In 1995 scientists at New York's Rockefeller University announced the discovery of a gene responsible for obesity in mice and humans. They argued it must be genes, not greed, that makes you fat and the next step is a pill that should guarantee weight-loss. This might take ten years or more, but it will be worth billions of pounds. If it works, and that is a big if, it will only affect a small percentage of people and end up giving false hope to thousands of others.

'One gene has been sequenced but we don't know yet if it will affect humans at all,' argues Dr Prentice. 'Scientists have found gene after gene in cancers but we are still nowhere near finding a cure for cancer. Less than a quarter of instances of obesity are due to genetics. Certainly fat people are more likely to have fat children but that is more often passed down by bad eating habits. From 1980–91, the number of clinically obese people in Britain doubled. All these people have the same genes they did before, so the increase in fatness has to be due to their habits. As a nation we spend 40% of our leisure time watching TV and there is far too much fat in our diets.'

Being fat is not like being short. You can look at someone and know when they are big and when they are obese. A mature adult cannot grow taller, that is an immutable fact. We are all victims of our genes but very few people are genetically doomed to be chronically obese. The rest of us can either give in or fight. Biologically, women are supposed to be pregnant all the time but through both chemical and physical contraception they have the option of taking control of their destinies. But this is not advocating body fascism – no one has to starve themselves, to be stick thin because that is what the fashion magazines demand. The stick insect has different problems from the obese individual, but the problem still comes from the head not the belly.

The only infallible way to lose weight is to eat less and exercise more.

You cannot 'spot reduce' fat content – reduce fat at will from hips and thighs. There is no exercise, magic cream, plastic wrap procedure, specific exercise programme or anything else other than liposuction, that will remove fat from a specific area. There are no quick fixes. Basically wherever you have the greatest gains in fat content is where you will lose it from first. So if you are losing weight, of course you will lose fat from those regions but it will also come off other places as well. Men generally store fat around their waist, while women generally keep it around their hips. That is usually the first place it builds up and it is the last place it will leave.

The best way to get, and keep, a washboard stomach, or shapely hips, is to follow a low fat diet and to do plenty of aerobic exercise. Crunches, or side leg raises, while strengthening and building the muscles, will not make them appear through the layer of fat between them and the skin. Get rid of the fat and a firm tummy will show up and the hips will become firm and trim.

We all have the only infallible diet mechanism, sitting on top of our shoulders – it's called a brain. It's the thing that controls our thought processes, that can provide the necessary motivation to challenge and change anything. If you are smart enough to want to get fit it is already working pretty well. What you choose to eat will help the process along.

CONTROLLING YOUR WEIGHT

The key to weight control is keeping energy intake (food) and energy output (physical activity) in balance. When you consume only as many calories as your body needs, your weight will usually remain constant. If you take in more calories than your body needs, you will put on excess fat. If you expend more energy than you take in, you will burn excess fat. Exercise plays an important role in weight control by increasing energy output, calling on stored calories for extra fuel. Recent studies show that not only does exercise increase metabolism during a workout, but it causes your metabolism to stay increased for a period of time after exercising, allowing you to burn more calories while you are recovering.

How much exercise is needed to make a difference in your weight depends on the amount and type of activity, and on how much you eat. Aerobic exercise burns body fat. A medium-sized adult would have to walk more than 30 miles to burn up 3,500 calories, the equivalent of one pound of fat. Although that may seem like a lot, you don't have to walk the 30 miles all at once. Walking a mile a day for 30 days will achieve the same result, providing you don't increase your food intake to negate the effects of walking. If you consume 100 calories a day more than your body needs, you will gain approximately 10lb in a year. You could take that weight off, or keep it off, by doing 30 minutes of moderate exercise daily.

The combination of exercise and diet offers the most flexible and effective approach to weight control. Since muscle tissue weighs more than fat tissue, and exercise develops muscle to a certain degree, your bathroom scale won't necessarily tell you whether or not you are 'fat'. Well-muscled individuals, with relatively little body fat, are invariably 'overweight' according to standard weight charts. If you are doing a regular programme of strength training, your muscles will increase in weight, and possibly your overall weight will increase. Body composition is a better indicator of your condition than body weight. Lack of physical activity causes muscles to get soft, and if food intake is not decreased, added body weight is almost always fat. Once-active people, who continue to eat as they always have after settling into sedentary lifestyles, tend to suffer from 'creeping obesity'.

But you have to continue to eat. Without food, our bodies slowly run down and eventually die. Food is more than a bulk that stops hunger, it is a fuel.

Body Fuel – What Makes Energy

In many ways the body runs like a motor car – one that is is never turned off but spends a lot of time idling in neutral. Both need fuel to function but use much less when idling, resting or simply sitting still. However, just as a car consumes much more petrol at 70 mph than it does at 55 mph, once your body starts to take strenuous exercise it needs more fuel. The muscles contract and stretch harder, the heart beats faster which pumps more blood around the body quicker and the lungs take in more oxygen. The body demands more energy. This energy comes from food and drink.

There are four components in food and drink that together produce energy: carbohydrates, fat, protein, alcohol. The digestive system breaks these down into different constituents which are then absorbed into the bloodstream. Carbohydrates are broken down into glucose, fructose and galactose; fats into fatty acids; protein into amino-acids while alcohol is absorbed directly into the blood. Carbohydrates and alcohol are used primarily to provide short-term energy, fats are a long term energy source while proteins are the reserve tank, producing energy in emergencies (when you have run out of carbohydrates) or recycling themselves into energy when they have reached the end of their useful life.

On paper, fat is the most concentrated form of energy, providing the body with more than twice as much energy as carbs and protein. 1g of carbohydrate or protein releases 4 kcal of energy, the same of alcohol 7 kcal and fat 9 kcal. After being converted into glycogen (it even sounds like rocket fuel), carbohydrate is stored in the muscles and the liver, along with three times its own weight of water. However the body can only store a certain amount of glycogen – about 1,600 kcal, which is enough to last you one day if you eat nothing. Fats are stored as adipose tissue all over the body, primarily around the organs and beneath the skin. Protein is used more as a building material rather than a fuel tank, it forms energy and organ tissue which can be broken down to release energy if necessary. The muscles and organs thus represent a potential source of energy.

Fuel Reserves in a 70kg (154lb) man – (potential energy available in kcal)

	Glycogen	Fats	Proteins
Liver	400	450	400
Adipose Tissue	0	135,000	0
Muscle	1,200	350	24,000

We haven't forgotten booze. Sadly, for all its high concentrated energy store, alcohol cannot be used as a fuel for exercise, no matter how bad the hangover or how hard the exercise. Only the liver has the specific enzymes to break down alcohol and it will only do this at a fixed pace. It doesn't take a genius to work out the equation: the more alcohol you consume the more weight you will put on.

During any form of physical activity, the body calls upon its energy sources in a different fuel mixture. Even at the end of a marathon, or other long strenuous exercise, protein only provides 10% of the fuel mixture. However just in case you are thinking of going on a low carbohydrate diet, thus depleting the glycogen reserves and forcing the body to eat up more fat don't bother. It doesn't work. The weight loss is initially water and then up to half from energy loss. It won't make you fitter, just weaker.

At rest, the body is burning 65%–80% fat, 20–35% glycogen. The body does this to conserve glycogen. It takes much less oxygen to burn glycogen than fat, and that is why the body's preferred fuel for heavy exercise is glycogen. It will replace the glycogen by further food intake or burning fat later on. The brain requires glycogen as it cannot burn fatty acids. If you are burning glycogen long enough the body realises that it is going to run out of glycogen pronto, so it shifts over to burning fatty acids to spare the glycogen supplies.

Visualize glycogen as rocket fuel, fat as diesel and your body as an engine that can take and mix them both together. During exercise the body naturally adjusts its fuel mixture to cope with the situation. The harder you exercise the more carbohydrates you use. When sprinting or taking part in other types of anaerobic activity hardly any energy will come from fat, it doesn't work fast enough. If you're trying to emulate a rocket you need rocket fuel. During a jog you will use both carbohydrate and fat, when you slow down from a faster to a slower pace you will burn a higher proportion of fat. Walking at a brisk pace you will be using diesel fuel; as soon as the pace increases more glycogen kicks in.

However, the longer you exercise aerobically the more the body strives to conserve its limited glycogen store. Unfortunately, it always requires a small amount of carbohydrate to break down fat, because fat never burns on its own. Looking at the fuel reserves chart above you can see that three-quarters of the body's supply of glycogen is stored in the muscles. Towards the end of endurance events the muscles will be depleted and it will call on the glycogen stored in the liver and start breaking down proteins to release amino-acids. After a very long period of continuous exercise the body can run out of glycogen, causing glucose levels in the blood to drop below normal. This can lead to hypoglycemia – fatigue, nausea and dizziness. This is a good time to stop exercising!

The more aerobic exercise you take the better your body becomes at getting the diesel/rocket fuel mix right. Fat starts to break down earlier in the session, sparing the glycogen store. If you start exercising after years of idleness your body will mainly rely on glycogen for the first 15–20 minutes of a session. Just as fat is starting to make a contribution to the fuel mixture you will feel too shattered to continue. An experienced athlete, on the other hand, will start burning fat much earlier, perhaps after a mere five minutes and be able to keep going for longer. Well-trained muscles develop the ability to store 20–50% more glycogen than untrained muscles. In 100g of muscle an untrained muscle will contain 13g of glycogen, a trained muscle 32g and special carbo-loading for endurance events can up this to 35–40g.

An unfit man or woman may have loads of potential energy bouncing around their bellies but if they don't have the glycogen reserves to help it combust nothing is going to happen. The lesson is simple. To exercise we must have a full tank of glycogen. How do we get it?

By eating a diet that is rich in carbohydrates.

WHAT'S IN FOOD?

As Geoff Hurst proved in that memorable World Cup Final, an athlete can perform to the height of his or her abilities on the 'wrong' diet. But most of us aren't that fit. We need as much help as we can get to give us the necessary edge, whether it be in developing the right exercise programme or following some basic dietary guidelines. Most people who live in the developed world eat a lot of the wrong stuff. Before you can plan what to eat you need to know what you are eating.

Food is composed of six nutrients:

CARBOHYDRATES

These are the little fellows that provide the primary energy source the body draws on when exercising hard and a source of the calories that fuel the muscles and the brain. High carbohydrate foods can be found in two basic kinds. One is starchy foods like pasta, wholewheat bread, cereals and pulses, which also contain other vitamins and minerals. The other is sugary foods in which the carbohydrates have been extracted and broken down so that they can be quickly absorbed into the digestive system. The disadvantage is that sweets, sugary drinks, and biscuits can also contain a lot of fat and very few other essential nutrients. If you are serious about training try to cut your sugar content in half.

Ideally, you should aim to replace foods rich in fat and sugar with low-fat foods. The body will continue to absorb energy from unprocessed food sources like potatoes, fruit and vegetables. This will also increase the intake of fibre which is good for the digestion. Carbohydrate is transformed into glycogen for use as fuel. You should aim to get 60–65% of the calories required from the starches and sugars found in carbohydrate-rich foods.

FATS

Fats are not quite the bad guys they are so often made out to be. Fats are an essential source of stored energy that we burn during low level activity – like reading and sleeping – and provide essential protection against the cold. We've made them the bad guys by eating too much and putting the wrong sort of fat in our diet. Fats are important sources of energy but the British probably consume too much for their own good. In other words, approach the great British cooked breakfast with caution, especially if you aren't taking enough exercise to burn it off. Saturated fats (generally taken from animals) can contribute to heart disease and some cancers, while unsaturated fats (primarily from vegetables) are less harmful, though no less calorie laden. Your eventual goal should be for only 25% of your daily diet to be fat.

PROTEIN

This is an important nutrient because it makes up part of the structure of every cell in the body. Three-quarters of the dry weight of human muscle is protein. Proteins are broken down in the gut into amino acids. All by itself, the body can make 12 of these, the other 8 must be obtained from the foods you eat every day. These 8 amino acids are called essential and are only found all together in animal products. Amino acids are required for building and repairing the components of tissues such as muscles, red blood cells, and hair and for synthesizing hormones. Under extreme conditions it is a source of calories which the body will use if there are inadequate carbs available. No matter what mummy told you, you don't have to eat animal protein (milk, cheese, yogurt, meat, poultry, fish and eggs) at every meal to survive. About 15% of your calories should come from protein-rich foods like fish, chicken and dried beans. Most of us eat much too much protein, and we would be well advised to follow the lead of other cultures who view protein more as a condiment on the dinner plate than the main attraction. Vegan vegetarians, who don't eat dairy or eggs, do nicely by choosing different plant proteins (rice, grain, cereals, nuts, seeds, dried beans and vegetables) that on their own are incomplete, but when combined provide all 8 essential amino acids.

VITAMINS

These are the metabolic catalysts that regulate the chemical reactions within the body. They include vitamins A, B complex, C, D, E and K. Generally they are chemical substances that the body does not manufacture itself so you must obtain them through diet. They do not provide energy. Signs of scurvy or other vitamin deficiencies are seldom seen in Western countries today. Recent surveys show that 30–80% of all athletes regularly take vitamin and mineral supplements, working on the assumption that if some vitamins are involved in energy metabolism, increasing the dosage will improve performance. However scientific findings suggest that this has no meaningful effect on performance. Just by eating a sensible variety of foods it is possible to get the necessary vitamins into the system. If you are on a very low calorie diet (see the 1,200 calorie menu planner in Body Food 2 page 167) we would advise taking a multivitamin supplement.

MINERALS

These elements are obtained from foods that combine in various ways to help form structures in the body – calcium in bones – or regulate bodily processes – iron in red blood cells helps transport oxygen. Other important minerals are magnesium, phosphorus, sodium, potassium and zinc. 5% of our body is made of minerals, and they are also essential to the maintenance of nerve and muscle function. It has become apparent that we do not know enough about the role and metabolism of minerals so the best advice is to make sure you get enough by eating a varied diet of unrefined foods. Iron is a major nutrient because of the vital role it plays in metabolism and the body's capacity to perform muscular work. Eat lots of beans, green leafy vegetables, whole grains with the occasional serving of liver (which tastes much better if you don't overcook it) and that should easily satisfy the body's requirements. Minerals do not provide energy either.

WATER

Water makes up 50–55% of your body weight. There are 75 pints of water in a healthy young man weighing 154lbs/70kg. Water keeps the body temperature stable, carries the nutrients to and waste away from cells and is needed to help the whole body system to function. It also helps control the body's temperature, as sweating during exercise results in the cooling of the body. Water does not provide energy. But do be aware that even small losses of water (2–3% loss of body weight) can seriously hinder performance. Stay hydrated!

GETTING THE RIGHT BALANCE

Okay, so how do I determine if I'm getting the right balance of nutrients in my food? The simplest way is to read the labels or to look at charts which show the nutrients available in food stuffs. The Recommended Dietary Allowance (RDA) is a standard for intake of nutrients which – as it is based on the requirements of growing teenage boys – meets or exceeds the needs of nearly everyone, including athletes.

Protein	65gs
Vitamin A	5,000 IU
Vitamin C	60mg
Thiamin	1.5mg
Riboflavin	1.7mg
Niacin	20mg
Calcium	1g
Iron	18mg
Vitamin D	400 IU

CARB POWER

Just in case you are dubious about the wondrous effects of carbohydrate-rich diets, there have been extensive scientific studies that have shown categorically that those who consume lots of carbs are able to exercise for longer. A study carried out at Loughborough University examined the effects of carbohydrate intake on running distances. Thirty subjects were asked to run to exhaustion at 70% VO2 max on a treadmill. There followed a three-day recovery period during which time the subjects were divided into three groups. In addition to their normal diets their energy intake was increased by 70% with either additional fat and protein (control group), or carbohydrate in the form of confectionery (confectionery group) or pasta, rice and potato (pasta group). The runners were then asked to repeat the exercise in an attempt to match or improve their original distances. The control group were only able to increase their average distance by 3% whereas the confectionery group and pasta group increased by 23% and 26%.

Athletes who have very high energy needs are familiar with the term 'carbo-loading' to describe the increased intake of carbohydrate food in the run-up to competition. This can easily be achieved by gradually reducing the amount of training during the week before competition, whilst increasing carbohydrate intake during the three to four days prior to competition. However carbo-loading is not recommended until you have achieved a high level of physical fitness.

So carbohydrates are good for you. They provide energy for exercise and have beneficial effects on the heart. But if you are aiming for 60–65% of your diet to be of carbohydrates, it's a good idea to know a little more about this source of fuel. Because most foods contain a variety of different nutrients it is easy to get confused by the spectrum of choice – refined versus wholemeal flours, honey or sugar and simple or complex carbohydrates.

Without going into excruciating technical detail, sugars – glucose, fructose and sucrose, table sugar, honey and the glucose polymers found in sports drinks – are simple carbohydrates which can provide energy without vitamins and minerals. Complex carbohydrates found in wholesome fruits, vegetables and grains provide energy with vitamins and minerals, all helping to fine tune the exercise engine.

Complex carbohydrates, or polysaccharides, are made mostly of strands of simple sugars which form long complex chains like strings of beads. They are found in grains, fruits, peas, beans, and other vegetables. Complex carbohydrates include three types of dietary fibre – cellulose, hemicellulose and gums – and starches. A single starch molecule may contain from 300 to 1,000 or more sugar units. The giant molecules are packed side by side in a plant root or seed, providing energy for the plant. All starches are plant materials. Cereal grains, such as wheat, rice and corn, are rich sources of starch, and constitute a large part of the world's food supply, generally in the form of breads and pastas. Starches are also found in potatoes and beans.

For a long time starchy foods were avoided by dieters as fattening, whereas in fact they are a good source of energy for those who want to lose weight. Many people think that starchy foods such as bread, potatoes and pasta are high in calories. They aren't – until you spread loads of butter on the bread, fill the baked potatoes with sour cream, and serve your pasta with a cream sauce. Remember that carbs (and proteins) provide only four calories per gram, while fat provides nine calories per gram. Without the toppings, or with only moderate amounts, complex carbohydrate foods can be less fattening than animal-protein foods that naturally contain fat.

It is no coincidence that complex carbohydrates provide the stuff of life in developing countries around the world. Potatoes were the staple crop for the peasants of Ireland and when they failed mass starvation followed. Without rice how would South East Asia feed itself? Potatoes, breads, cereals, and other foods high in complex carbohydrates have always been regarded as cheap and essential – the survival crop for the poor. But carbo-hydrate-rich diets are also good for you. High fat diets have been linked to heart disease and some cancers, protein-rich meals are no longer considered the lunch of World Cup champions. High dietary fibre (found mostly in complex carbohy-drates) is reported to possibly reduce the risk of colon cancer and heart disease, and as we learn that a five-ounce steak has more calories than an equal amount of bread, pasta or pota-toes (hold the butter), complex carbohydrates are becoming the chosen food of the rich and middle classes, too.

So eating carbohydrates is not just good for your glycogen supplies, it has other long terms benefits for your whole body. It can help weight loss, reduce the risk of heart disease and improve your all-round health.

A diet high in carbohydrates may be more slimming than a diet of comparable calories that is high in fat. A research report published in the January 1989 *American Journal of Clinical Nutrition* suggested that 'altering the composition of the diet in favour of a higher carbohydrate-to-fat ratio may decrease the incidence of obesity'. The researchers also found that when the participants switched to a diet high in complex carbohydrates, they became full more quickly and thus uncon-sciously decreased their intake of calories. When you cut down on fat, the high fibre, complex carbohydrates found in fruits, vegetables and whole grains, fill you up without filling you out.

Adding more fibre to your diet means that you must drink more fluids. If you don't, you'll become constipated which could be an excuse to revert to your old dietary habits.

Along with starches, fibre – the other important category of complex carbohydrates – is also gaining popularity for health reasons. Like starches, dietary fibre is found abundantly in plants, especially in the outer layers of cereal grains and the fibrous parts of fruits, beans, and other vegetables. Eating foods high in fibre has been found to reduce symptoms of chronic constipation, diverticular disease and some types of irritable bowel syndrome while there is some indication that plant fibre may reduce blood pressure. It has also been suggested that diets low in fibre may increase the risk of developing colon cancer. These effects emphasize the importance of whole grains, dried beans and peas, carrots, and other once overlooked sources of complex carbohydrates.

Where do I look for a good source of starch and fibre?

Complex Carbohydrates
Breads, both wholegrain and white (wholegrain will contain more minerals and vitamins)
Breakfast cereals, cooked and ready-to-eat
Flours, wholegrain and white
Pastas, such as macaroni and spaghetti
Barley and rice
Noodles
Pulses – dried peas, beans and lentils
Potatoes, yams, sweet potatoes and eddoes
Plantains (green bananas)
Parsnips
Sweetcorn
Snacks high in Carbohydrates
Bananas (wonder food for athletes, high in potassium as well)
Raisins
Other dried fruit
Confectionery (though watch out for too much sugar and fats – read the labels)
Sweetened yogurt
Muesli bars
Fruit juice
Sports drinks

Simple Carbohydrates
Sugar (white and brown)
Jam, honey and other preserves
Sweets, chocolates and other confectionery
Cakes and biscuits
Puddings and desserts
Fruit yogurt and other dairy desserts
Sweet pastries and pies
Ice cream, custard and jelly
Soft drinks
Sweet pickles and sauces
Fruit
Milk
Fruit juices
Wine
Beer

Most simple carbohydrates, with the exception of juices are empty calorie foods. Because they don't contain any fibre, they enter your bloodstream quickly. It feels great when the sugar is going in, but two hours later, when you come off the sugar high, you either feel lousy and live through it, or you reach for more sugar. Then you feel lousy again and repeat the cycle. Try to consume no more than 10% of your total calories from simple carbohydrate foods.

HOW MUCH CARBOHYDRATE DO I NEED TO MUNCH IN A DAY TO GET THE MAXIMUM BENEFITS ?

Aim for a minimum of 60–65% of your diet to be carbohydrates. 55% of your total calorie intake should be complex carbohydrates.

Average Daily Calorie Intake	Carbohydrate Needed to Give 60% of Calories
1,500	225g
2,000	300g
2,500	375g
3,000	450g
3,500	525g
4,000	600g

To help you further the list below sets out the amount of different foods needed to obtain 50g of carbohydrate. Please note that not all of them are complex carbohydrates.

500ml soft drink
3 medium-sized apples
600ml fruit juice (1 pint)
1 litre milk (skimmed or semi-skimmed)
50g sugar (try sprinkling it over things)
100g crisps/corn chips
325g baked beans
150g boiled wholemeal rice
200g boiled pasta (covered in tomato sauce, hold the cream !)
Half 9in-base pizza (add low fat mozzarella and vegetable toppings for extra carbs)
2 average helpings of porridge (made with semi-skimmed milk)
5 wholewheat biscuits
3 bananas
8 rice cakes
5 rice cakes with 1 banana
4/5 slices bread
1 jacket potato (175g)
10 cream crackers
6 plain crackers or crispbreads with 1tbsp. of jam/honey/marmalade or 2tbsp pure fruit spread
5 fig rolls
75–90g chocolate-covered snack bar (beware the sugar highs and lows)

FATS

Like most everybody else in the Western World you are probably battered with all the information about fats. You can't live with them and you can't live without them. One moment saturated animal fats are killing people left right and centre, the next reports from France seem to indicate that peasants eating lots of rich fatty food cooked in goose fat and drinking red wine live longer than born-again vegetarian fitness fanatics. However, as the government survey quoted earlier in the chapter shows, we are getting more obese as a nation by the year. Excess saturated fat, cholesterol refined foods and gooey calorie heavy puddings contribute substantially to problems like obesity, heart disease, cancer, diabetes, hypertension, kidney failure and other diseases of aging. Simply increasing your carbohydrate intake at the expense of fats will not only fuel your engine for better mileage, it will also help cut down the number of services required.

There are two types of fat, saturated and unsaturated (see the chart below). Saturated fat is the one that does the most damage to your body. The unsaturated fats also have two categories: polyunsaturated and monounsaturated. It's easy to recognize most saturated fat because it is solid at room temperature. Foods composed of or cooked with saturated fats raise the blood cholesterol level, which in turn increases the risk of heart disease. The exceptions to this are the tropical oils, palm and coconut, hydrogenated fat and margarine. Tropical oils are found mostly in baked goods; hydrogenated fats are found mostly in margarine. We recommend eating mostly monounsaturated fats, such as olive, canola, and avocado oil. Monounsaturated fats found in olive oil and canola are particularly good for protecting the heart and have more flavour. Use olive oil for salad dressings and groundnut (peanut oil) for cooking. The next best choices are the polyunsaturated fats, such as soybean, safflower, corn, and sesame seed oil. Good or bad, be aware that they all contain the same amount of calories per gram!

Fat	Saturated	Monounsaturated	Polyunsaturated
Coconut oil	90%	10%	0%
Palm oil	50	30	20
Butter	65	30	5
Beef fat	50	45	5
Chicken fat	30	50	20
Olive oil	15	75	10
Canola oil	5	60	35
Groundnut oil	20	50	30
Safflower oil	10	15	75
Sunflower oil	10	20	70
Corn oil	15	25	60
Cottonseed oil	25	20	55

HOW DO I SET ABOUT CUTTING DOWN MY FAT INTAKE?

Your aim is to have no more than 20–25% of your diet as fat. Take it slowly because it is not going to be that easy. So much of the food we buy has got fat in it. Take another look at that list of Simple Carbohydrates. Most of them seemed pretty appetising at the time – the problem is that a great many processed foods are also full of fats.

If you are serious you will need to start studying food labels and start doing some simple maths. Remember that 1g fat = 9 calories (to make calculations a little easier round that up to 10 calories) and 1g protein or carbohydrates = 4 calories. Now look again at those encouraging '95% fat-free' labels. Look carefully at how many calories come from fat. If something has 120 calories, which is pretty low, but it has 9g fat and 5g protein and 5g carbohydrates, almost 70% of that product is fat. Try to eliminate the fat that you eat. There is fat in virtually everything so aiming for a zero fat diet will probably put you in the 10–20% class, just because not everything is fat free, and you do need some fat in your diet.

Cutting down on fat intake is easier than it sounds. Look at it this way. One pound of fat provides 3,500 calories, so you need to eat 3,500 calories less than normal to lose a pound of a fat – taken over a week that is only 500 calories a day, or a six-ounce burger one day, and two chocolate bars the next. Start by eating less of the following: butter, margarine and other spreading fats, fried foods, greasy hamburgers, sausages, hot dogs, pastries, cakes, biscuits, chocolate, crisps and fast food snacks.

The next step is to switch to low fat alternatives: skimmed or semi-skimmed milk, low fat yogurts, low fat spreads for bread, lean cuts of meat, chicken or turkey (but make sure you remove the skin before cooking) and more fish (just make sure the fish isn't cooked in batter!). White fish like cod and plaice are extremely low in fat, while oily fish like mackerel and salmon are known to be very good for the heart. Repeat after me: carbohydrates are not fattening.

Remember that if you have gone on a low fat diet you will have reduced your calorie intake substantially. If you are simultaneously increasing the level of your exercise programme that may leave you feeling weaker, because you have not fully replenished the glycogen fuel supplies in your muscles. It is something to be aware of, but is also easily remedied. Where you used to eat one baked potato covered in lashings of butter or sour cream, now eat two baked potatoes with a smidgen of low fat spread.

PROTEIN

Just when sports nutritionists thought it was all over, the protein debate has sprung back into life. Back in the 1960s it was thought that what an athlete needed was lashings of protein – platefuls of beef, tuna, eggs and chicken which would help build muscles the size of the Himalayas. As protein is the major constituent of muscles this seemed perfectly logical. Then research switched the other way, suggesting that an athlete needed no more protein than anyone else and that carbohydrates were the answer. In the last ten years new research indicates that the protein needs of strength and endurance athletes may be higher than believed.

Weight-lifters have long held true to building muscle through protein, while runners favour carbohydrates at the expense of protein consumption. Professional athletes tend to develop individual idiosyncrasies so we aren't going to get involved, beyond diplomatically suggesting that you need to find a balance. A high protein diet will not lead to increased strength and bigger muscles by itself – you have to exercise those muscles hard as well. The most important thing is to get your priorities right.

What the body needs is enough energy to perform. Only when its needs have been met can it deal with other functions such as muscle growth and repair. In one study, the protein breakdown was measured in athletes after an hour of exercise.

It was considerably higher in athletes on low-carbohydrate diets. If the diet does not include enough carbohydrate the body will start breaking down muscle to keep on going. That is not what you want.

Research shows that the body breaks down protein fastest during and after exercise. At the same time the manufacture of protein slows down. The longer the session the more protein is broken down. The more intense the session the more protein is broken down. Exercise acts as a trigger to activate one enzyme that oxidizes certain essential amino acids. So if you do eat enough protein to compensate for that loss or you overtrain, thus giving the body no chance to replenish its stores, the net result will be a loss of muscle which will affect your performance.

HOW MUCH PROTEIN DO I NEED?

It's easy to calculate how much protein you need. First identify yourself in this protein intake chart (it already includes a margin of safety for growing teenagers and body builders).

Category	Grams of protein/pound of body weight
Sedentary adult	0.4
Active adult	0.4–0.6
Growing athlete	0.6–0.9
Adult building muscle mass	0.6–0.9

Now multiply your weight in pounds by the number for your category to give you the number of grams of protein you need each day. A 10-stone (140lb) athletic woman would need about 84g of protein a day – the same requirement as a 15-stone (210lb) male office worker whose only exercise is going to watch the football every Saturday.

It's easy to keep track of your protein intake – all it takes is a little time. List everything you eat and drink for a minimum of one 24-hour period. Then use the nutritional information on the food labels to show you how much protein you have consumed. A can of skipjack tuna might tell you it contains 25g of protein per serving and two servings per can. If you scoffed the lot in one sitting you got 50g of protein and if you are that

10-stone athletic woman then you have had 60% of your recommended intake in one meal. Here are some other protein values for food stuffs that may not be labelled:

THE PROTEIN VALUE OF VARIOUS FOODS

Quantity/Food	Protein(g)
1 pint (600ml) skimmed milk	19.3
2oz (50g) cheddar cheese	12.8
8.8oz (250g) cottage cheese	34.5
5.4oz (150g) yogurt	7.7
6oz (175g) lean steak	48.3
6oz (175g) chicken	38.2
6oz (175g) cod	30.5
2 large eggs	14
1 small potato	2
8oz (225g) baked beans	11.5
8oz (225g) cooked lentils	17.1
2oz (50g) peanuts	12.2
2 slices wholemeal bread	6.4
6oz (175g) steamed rice	4.6

If you want a rule of thumb for getting adequate, but not excess protein in your diet, aim to have 2 cups of low fat milk or yogurt (do not forget that many protein rich foods are also high in fat and choose the low fat alternatives) plus 4–6oz (100–175g) of protein-rich foods per day. Combined with the extra little amounts of protein in the other foods that you eat that should provide for all your needs.

Breakfast: one cup semi-skimmed milk on cereal
Lunch: 2oz (50g) protein sandwich filling (tuna, chicken, turkey, lean beef)
       Yogurt
Dinner: 4oz (100g) meat, fish, poultry or equivalent in pulses

Don't forget that you need to eat other foods rich in (yes, you guessed it) carbohydrates, to round out your daily nutritional requirements.

CHOLESTEROL

While we are on the subject of diet it is very important – especially for men – to look out for your cholesterol levels. Heart disease is a major killer in this country but even if you have a history of heart disease in the family your destiny is in your hands. Obviously increasing your level of aerobic exercise will help but so will changing your diet. No matter what your age, if you change your dietary habits, you will see benefits. If you maintain your ideal body weight and stop smoking, you're headed in the right direction.

WHAT ARE THE RISK FACTORS FOR HEART DISEASE?

- Are you overweight?
- Do you smoke?
- Are you under a lot of stress?
- Do you have high blood pressure?
- Do you eat a high-fat diet? Especially one that is high in saturated fat.
- Do you know your blood cholesterol level and have you had the test done to determine how much is good and bad?

Cholesterol is a waxy substance that contributes to hardening of the arteries. It accumulates on the walls of blood vessels throughout the body, especially in the heart. This build-up contributes to heart attacks by limiting blood flow to the heart. There are two types of cholesterol. HDL (high density lipoprotein) is the good guy because it helps carry the bad stuff out of the arteries. Because exercise tends to boost HDL, active people have a higher percentage of it, and the higher the percentage of HDL the lower the risk of heart problems. LDL (low density lipoprotein) is the bad stuff that causes clogging and blocking of the arteries. At least 25% of your total cholesterol should therefore be HDL cholesterol.

In America, the National Institute of Health recommend that

all adults over the age of 20 have a cholesterol test every five years. If that level is high it should then be re-measured looking at both HDL levels and total cholesterol.

Here are the guidelines for blood cholesterol levels. Do you know where you stand?

	Desirable	Increased Risk	Higher Risk
Total cholesterol	<200 mg/dl	200–239 mg/dl	240 or greater mg/dl
LDL (bad cholesterol)	<130 mg/dl	130–159 mg/dl	160 or greater mg/dl
Triglycerides	<200 mg/dl	200–400 mg/dl	400 or greater mg/dl
HDL (good cholesterol)	>35 mg/dl	<35 mg/dl	<35 mg/dl

Note: mg/dl = the number of mg of cholesterol per 100cc of blood.

The ratio of Total Cholesterol: HDL is an indicator of the risk of heart disease. The ratio should be less than 4 to 1.
For example: Total Cholesterol: HDL Example 200: 50 = 4:1

While cholesterol plays many roles in the body, you don't have to eat it, because your liver can make all that the body needs. Try to consume less than 300mg a day. It's only present in foods from animal sources (dairy, eggs, meat, fish and poultry), plants do not contain cholesterol. Therefore, don't be fooled by the advertisements saying that cholesterol was removed from foods made from plants – there wasn't any there to begin with! But just because a food doesn't have cholesterol, the label doesn't say anything about whether or not it contains saturated fat! You have to read the labels.

Do you know how much cholesterol is in some of your favourite foods?

Cholesterol Levels in Selected Foods

Food	Amount	Cholesterol (mg)
Milk, skim fluid	1 cup	4
Milk, dry whole	100g	85
Milk 2%	1 cup	18
Milk, whole	1 cup	34
Cheese		
Cheddar	1oz (25g)	30
Cottage, creamed	½ cup	17
Cream	100g	120
Ice Cream	½ cup	30
Beef, lamb, pork (lean)	3oz (75g)	77–79
Veal	3oz	129
Liver	3oz	270
Sweetbreads, kidneys	3oz	329
Heart	3oz	164
Brains	3oz	1746
Chicken	3oz	72–80
Turkey	3oz	60–72
Salmon	3oz	74
Tuna, canned in water	3oz	55
Halibut	3oz	55
Clams	3oz	55
Crab	3oz	85
Lobsters	3oz	70
Oysters	3oz	92
Scallops	3oz	35
Shrimp	3oz	130
Egg, whole	One	208
Egg Yolk	One	208
Egg White	One	0
Mayonnaise	1tbsp	10
Butter	1tbsp	11

JEREMY'S TRAINING TIP
DIET AND FOOD

At one stage the England team were being advised on precisely what to eat, what was good, what was bad, how much it should weigh and so on. It was very precise and I found it very hard to be so disciplined. Fortunately the diet I like is conducive to what I do – lots of carbohydrates, a lot of chicken and pasta. I didn't used to like vegetables but as I get older I find I do enjoy them. I would never eat too many bad things but I love chocolate, and chips I'm just crazy about, so I was never going to give them up. For me it is about listening to the body, not slavishly following a diet. Every now and then if I feel a bit low, a bit tired, I get checked out for iron deficiency, which is a good excuse to pop down the pub and have a couple of pints of Guinness. Sally will have a couple of beers, a chocolate bar or a packet of crisps if she fancies them but generally she eats very well. We are very lucky as athletes that we train so hard and so the odd indulgence we may have goes unnoticed because the body burns it away. The lesson is that if you train hard you can afford to reward yourself every now and again.

QUESTIONS

1. An average can of Cola contains the equivalent of how many teaspoons of sugar, is it 1, 3 or 5?
2. Olive oil contains less fat than corn oil. True or false?
3. What percentage of the calories in normal mayonnaise are provided by fat – 30%, 50% or 99%
4. Which contains the most calories, one tablespoon of normal mayonnaise or three chocolate digestives?
5. How many calories per ounce does sugar contain – 60, 110 or 170 calories?
6. Does plain or milk chocolate have the highest sugar content?
7. We all need a certain amount of salt each day, but how much – 2,800, 4,100 or 4,600mg?
8. Which organ regulates the level of salt in the human body?
9. Protein has how many calories per gram, 4, 7 or 9?
10. Carbohydrate has how many calories per gram, 4, 6 or 9?
11. Fat has how many calories per gram, 4, 9 or 12?
12. How much is the recommended dietary allowance for cholesterol in milligrams a day: no more than 300, 400 or 500?

(Answers at the end of the book)

CHAPTER 13

BODY FOOD 2: WHAT TO EAT FOR EXERCISE

WHEN DO I EAT DURING AN EXERCISE PROGRAMME?

There has been some debate about the effects of carbohydrate intake immediately before and during exercise. Some athletes believe that eating carbohydrate before exercise reduces performance, but recent scientific studies have disproved this.

Solid carbohydrate in the form of a chocolate bar has been shown to improve cycling performance when eaten in small amounts throughout exercise. In a study carried out at Ball State University, Indiana, USA, ten men were given a confectionery snack at hourly intervals during a four-hour cycling exercise. On another occasion they repeated the exercise with a sugar-free drink instead of the confectionery. In a sprint ride to exhaustion at the end of the exercise, the subjects were able to cycle 45% longer when confectionery was taken than when the sugar-free control drink was taken. However bear in mind that a large intake of simple carbohydrates can lead to sugar highs, followed by a crash later.

Although the need for a high carbohydrate intake is well recognized among endurance athletes, sprinters and games players often fail to appreciate that their muscle glycogen stores may be substantially depleted in training as well as in competition and must be replaced. Athletes who train intensively for 60–90 minutes expend as much as 1,000–1,400 kcals. If they wish to replace their muscle glycogen concentrations on a daily basis then they may need to increase their carbohydrate intake by as much as 500g. This is well within the dietary capacity of men, but not women, since this amount can equal their total energy intake. A practical rule, for both men and women, is to eat 7–10g of carbohydrates per kg of body weight per day during intense training.

Glycogen is restored to the muscles at a rate of about 5% per hour. Thus it takes at least 20 hours to fully replenish stocks. During the first 2 hours after exercise, glycogen is restored at a faster rate – 7% – as the body is desperate to refuel. Nutritionists therefore recommend that athletes eat or drink carbohydrates as soon after exercise as is practical to ensure that maximum restoration is taking place. However don't stuff yourself with a huge bowl of pasta immediately after exercise as your stomach might have an instant violent reaction. Frequent, smaller meals are probably better than large carbohydrate meals, so there's no need to go nuts (though you can have a handful of nuts if you want). Eat 50–100g of carbohydrate every 2 hours – little and often seems to be the rule.

Sports nutritionists firmly believe that breakfast is the most important meal of the day. Yes, mother was right all along. However if she believed that a hearty breakfast should consist of fried eggs, bacon, fried bread, toast smothered in butter and mugs of tea with eight sugars she was also mistaken. That is a recipe for heart disease. Your breakfast should be designed to replenish energy levels for the day ahead but not to stuff you so your body feels leaden. (See page 171 for some low calorie but nourishing breakfasts.)

The commonest excuses for skipping breakfast are 'I just don't have the time' and 'I'm not hungry in the morning'. And that is what they are – excuses. It's not difficult to grab a wholemeal roll, a yogurt and a banana on the way to work. If you are not hungry in the morning it's often because you ate too much last night – perhaps those biscuits while watching the movie were not such a good idea.

DIETARY GUIDELINES

Here are some basic dietary guidelines to follow. We will get into specifics later in the chapter.

■ Eat a variety of foods to get the energy (calories), protein, vitamins, minerals, and fibre you need for good health.
■ Balance the food you eat with physical activity. Maintain or improve your weight to reduce your chances of having high blood pressure, heart disease, a stroke, certain cancers, and the most common kind of diabetes.
■ Choose a diet low in fat, particularly saturated fat, and cholesterol to reduce risk of heart disease and certain types of cancer. Because fat contains more than twice the calories of an equal amount of carbohydrate or protein, a diet low in fat can help you maintain a healthy weight.
■ Choose a diet with plenty of grain products, vegetables and fruits that provide much-needed vitamins, minerals, fibre, and complex carbohydrates. They are generally lower in fat.
■ Choose a diet moderate in sugars, salt and sodium. A diet with lots of sugar has too many calories and too few nutrients for most people and can contribute to tooth decay. A diet high in salt and sodium can contribute to high blood pressure, heart disease and stroke.
■ If you drink alcohol, do so in moderation. Alcoholic drinks supply calories, but little or no nutrients. Drinking alcohol is also the cause of many health problems and accidents and can lead to addiction. If you do consume alcohol, moderation is defined as no more than one drink a day for women and two drinks a day for men. One drink is considered to be 12oz of beer, 5oz of wine or 1.5oz of 80-proof distilled spirits.

Balance, variety and moderation are important concepts to keep in mind:

■ Balance includes an appropriate number of servings from each of the five main food groups each day.

- Variety means enjoying a number of different foods within any given food group, rather than having the same foods day after day. Variety makes meals more interesting and helps ensure a diet with sufficient vitamins and minerals.
- Moderation gives limits, but don't necessarily eliminate foods with excess fats, oils and sugars. If you practice balance and variety with the five main food groups, it will also help keep your intake of fats and sugars within reasonable limits.

In a word? Eat sensibly (okay, that's two words).
Here are some tips.

- Food does not come ready packaged with a big label saying 'masses of carbohydrates' or 'loadsafat'. There is no super magic food; each one offers its own unique brand of nutrients. For example, oranges are rich in vitamin C and carbohydrates but contain no iron or protein. Variety is not just the spice but the key to successful eating habits.
- Eaten in moderation snack attack foods, fizzy drinks and crisps can fit into your diet. No one food by itself is a junk food, but lots quzzled one after the other quickly makes it a junk food diet. You have to balance the sugar rush and fat attack caused by eating a chocolate bar with a simple low fat wholemeal chicken sandwich at the next meal. Wherever possible choose natural or lightly processed foods. Natural foods have more nutritional value and fewer dodgy additives. So choose whole-wheat not white bread, apples not apple juice, and baked potatoes not a bag of chips.
- You don't have to eat three square meals a day to have a well-rounded diet. Choose a selection of wholesome grub from the five major food groups: dairy, fruits, vegetables, meats and protein alternates, grains and cereals. Each foodstuff provides a different proportion of vitamins of minerals. Selecting from 1,200–1,500 calories a day from these foods, you can easily consume the RDA of the nutrients other than calories you need for a healthy diet.
- Don't be fooled by advertising claims. Read the labels in the

food you buy. It may sound like a chore but it can be very educational. Don't assume that a can of soup has a calorie count based on the whole can. Watch out for how many servings there are. The information on the label is based on a serving and you can be easily fooled.

START WITH THE STAPLES

If you understand the basics then it's time to stock up at home and make sure that temptation is easy to overcome. This is a list of basic foods that don't spoil quickly and can be pulled together to provide a healthy meal at any time of day. Most are also quite cheap!

Cupboard	Fridge	Freezer
Spaghetti	Light cheese spread	Wholemeal rolls
Rice	Parmesan cheese	Pitta bread
Wheat noodles	Low fat cottage cheese	Multigrain bread
Potatoes	Low fat yogurt	Orange juice concentrate
Crackers/crispbread	Semi-skimmed milk	Broccoli
Tomato pasta sauce	Eggs	Spinach
Canned tuna	Carrots	Chicken
Canned salmon	V–8 juice	Extra lean mince
Kidney beans	Onions	Ground turkey
Lentils	Low fat spread	Frozen fish (mackerel)
Peanut butter	Mushrooms	
Bran flakes	Garlic	
Oat bran	Tomatoes	
Muesli	Green beans	
Raisins/dried fruit		

WHAT COUNTS AS ONE SERVING?

Try to stick to one serving of any foodstuffs high in fat when eating a meal and make up with extra from high carbohydrate foods. It may not look like much to begin with, but the body quickly becomes accustomed to it.

BREAD, CEREAL, RICE AND PASTA

1 slice bread; ½ hamburger roll, bagel or English muffin; 3–4 plain crackers; ½ cup cooked cereal, rice or pasta; 1oz (25g) ready-to-eat cereal

VEGETABLES

½ cup chopped raw or cooked vegetables; 1 cup leafy raw vegetables; ¾ cup vegetables juice

FRUITS

1 piece of whole fruit or melon wedge; ½ cup canned, chopped or cooked fruit; ¼ cup dried fruit; ¾ cup juice

MILK, YOGURT AND CHEESE

1 cup milk or yogurt; 1½ – 2oz (40–50g) cheese

MEAT, POULTRY, FISH, DRY BEANS, EGGS AND NUTS

2½–3oz (65–75g) cooked lean meat, poultry or fish. Count ½ cup cooked beans, or 1 egg, or 2 tablespoons peanut butter as 1oz lean meat.

FATS, OILS, AND SWEETS

Limit calories from these, especially if you need to lose weight.

And while we are on the subject of charts and tables, here is a chart based on the Top Ten foodstuffs for athletes in training that might help with menu planning. It also shows why the basic staples you just bought are good for you:

TOP TEN CHART:
(Based on 100 grams of foodstuff, all figures in grams except for calories. T= trace)

Food	Protein	Fat	Fibre	Carbo-hydrates	Calories
Pasta	15.2	3	0	65	347
Oats	12.4	8.7	7	72	400
Bread	8.8	2.7	8.5	41.8	216
Beans	22	1.7	25	45	270
Yogurt	5	low	none	6.2	52
Dried fruit	8	0	none	64.4	240
Potatoes	1.2	T	2	18	120
Fish (tuna)	28	6	none	none	185
Bananas	1	T	2	10	110
Mushrooms	4	T	2	30	4

MENU PLANNING

You've made up your mind and you've committed to eating a certain number of calories a day – so where do you go from here? It's not always easy to figure out what a certain number of calories looks like when they're parcelled out over three meals and a snack during the day. If you look at the tables below, you can see just how to eat those calories, and stay healthy. Please note that if you choose to eat only 1,200 calories a day, you should consider taking a multivitamin to be sure that you are getting your minimum daily requirements of vitamins and minerals.

This is a good menu to prove to yourself that you don't need to eat so much. Men in particular should not stay on this menu for too long if they are exercising heavily.

SAMPLE MEAL PLAN – 1,200 CALORIES

Breakfast

Food Item	Portion	Calories	Protein	Carbs	Fat	Sodium
Egg whites omelette	½ cup	60	12	2	0	200
Mixed vegetables	1 cup	107	5	24	0.3	64
Wholewheat toast	1 slice	86	4	16	1.5	172
Jam/preserves	1 tbsp.	16	0	4	0	8
Black coffee	1 cup	5	0	1	0	0
Total		**274**	**21**	**47**	**1.8**	**444**

Lunch

Food Item	Portion	Calories	Protein	Carbs	Fat	Sodium
White meat turkey	3oz (75g)	119	26	0	3	48
Mustard	2 tsp.	8	0.5	0.6	0.5	130
Lettuce leaves	2	5	0.4	1	0	4
Cress	¼ cup	2	0.3	0.3	0	0.5
Wholewheat bread	2 slices	172	7	32	3	344
Total		**306**	**34.2**	**33.9**	**6.5**	**412.5**

Dinner

Food Item	Portion	Calories	Protein	Carbs	Fat	Sodium
Pasta	1.5 cups	284	10	57	1.3	2
Tomato sauce	½ cup	85	2	13	4	550
Steamed string beans	1 cup	44	2	10	0.3	4
Mixed salad	2 cups	50	2.5	10	0.7	28
Nonfat salad dressing	2 tbsp.	50	0	11	0	270
Water	16oz	0	0	0	0	0
Total		**513**	**16.5**	**101**	**6.3**	**860**

Snack

Food Item	Portion	Calories	Protein	Carbs	Fat	Sodium
Apple, medium	one	80	0.3	21	0.5	0
Grand Total		**1173**	**72**	**202.9**	**15.1**	**1830.5**

SAMPLE MEAL PLAN – 1,650 CALORIES

Breakfast

Food Item	Portion	Calories	Protein	Carbs	Fat	Sodium
Cheerios	2 cups	178	7	31	3	491
Semi-skimmed milk	1 cup	102	8	12	3	123
Whole wheat toast	1 slice	86	4	16	1.5	172
Apple butter	1 tbsp.	33	0	9	0	0
Banana	1	105	1	27	0.5	1
Black coffee	1 cup	5	0	1	0	0
Total Beakfast		**509**	**20**	**96**	**8**	**787**

Lunch

Food Item	Portion	Calories	Protein	Carbs	Fat	Sodium
Minestrone soup	1 cup	79	4	12	2	495
Tuna in brine	3 oz (75g)	99	22	0	0.7	288
Mayonnaise – fat free	2 tbsp.	21	0	5	0	338
Lettuce leaves	2	5	0.4	1	0	4
Tomato	half	13	0.5	3	0.2	6
Wholewheat bread	2 slices	172	7	32	3	0.5
Pear	1	98	0.6	25	0.6	0
Sparkling water	2 cups	0	0	0	0	0
Total Lunch		**487**	**34.5**	**78**	**6.5**	**1131.5**

Dinner

Food Item	Portion	Calories	Protein	Carbs	Fat	Sodium
Chicken	1 breast	167	25	0	6.6	70
Baked potato	1 med.	133	3	31	0	10
Low-cal. sour cream	2 tbsp.	41	1	1	4	12
Green beans	1 cup	44	2	10	0	4
Mixed lettuce	2 cups	50	2.5	10	0.7	28
Nonfat dressing	2 tbsp.	50	0	11	0	270
Water	10 oz	0	0	0	0	0
Total Dinner		**485**	**33.5**	**63**	**11.3**	**394**

Snack

Food Item	Portion	Calories	Protein	Carbs	Fat	Sodium
Popcorn	1 bag	150	4	22	2	340
Grand Total		**1631**	**92**	**259**	**27.8**	**2652.5**

SAMPLE MEAL PLAN – 2,000 CALORIES

Breakfast

Food Item	Portion	Calories	Protein	Carbs	Fat	Sodium
Bagel, 3oz, plain	one	234	9	45	1	454
Cream cheese, low fat	2 tbsp.	69	3	2	5	89
Grapefruit	half	37	0.7	9	0	0
Black coffee	1 cup	5	0	1	0	0
Total Breakfast		**345**	**12.7**	**57**	**6**	**543**

Lunch

Food Item	Portion	Calories	Protein	Carbs	Fat	Sodium
Flour tortilla/pita bread	one	115	3	20	2.5	169
Black beans	half cup	113	8	20	0.5	0.9
Spanish rice	half cup	108	2	21	2	162
Lettuce, chopped	¼ cup	2	0	0	0	1
Tomato, chopped	half	13	0.5	3	0	6
Onion, chopped	2 tbsp	8	0.2	2	0	0.6
Salsa/Mexican	¼ cup	12	0.5	3	0	234
Apple, medium	one	80	0.3	21	0.5	0
Milk, non-fat	1 cup	85	8	12	0	126
Total Lunch		**536**	**22.5**	**102**	**5.5**	**699.5**

Dinner

Food Item	Portion	Calories	Protein	Carbs	Fat	Sodium
Salmon, grilled	3oz (75g)	121	17	0	5.4	45
Olive oil	1 tsp.	45	0	0	5	0
Brown rice, long grain	1 cup	216	5	45	2	10
Mixed vegetables	1 cup	107	5	24	0.3	64
Tossed green salad	2 cups	50	2.5	10	0.7	28
Tomato. medium	3 slices	13	0.5	3	0	5
Cucumber, with peel	6 slices	3	0.2	0.6	0	0.5
Low fat dressing	3 tbsp.	45	2	1	3	552
Wholewheat roll	1 small	131	4	25	1.3	261
Butter	1 tsp	34	0	0	4	39
Water	16oz	0	0	0	0	0
Total Dinner		**765**	**36.2**	**108.6**	**21.7**	**1004.5**

Snacks

Food Item	Portion	Calories	Protein	Carbs	Fat	Sodium
Yogurt, nonfat, fruit	8oz	115	10	18	0.4	90
Raisins	50g	145	2.1	69.3	0.4	60
Total Snacks		**260**	**12.1**	**87.3**	**0.8**	**150**
Grand Total		**1906**	**83.5**	**354.9**	**34**	**2397**

SAMPLE MEAL PLAN – 2,500 CALORIES

Breakfast

Food Item	Portion	Calories	Protein	Carbs	Fat	Sodium
Waffles, low fat	two	160	6	32	1	560
Pancake syrup, light	4 tbsp.	100	0	26	0	180
Bacon, grilled	2 pieces	87	11	0.6	4	727
Strawberries	1 cup	43	0.9	10	0.5	1
Milk, nonfat	1 cup	85	8	12	0	126
Black coffee	1 cup	5	0	1	0	0
Total Breakfast		**480**	**25.9**	**81.6**	**5.5**	**1594**

Lunch

Food Item	Portion	Calories	Protein	Carbs	Fat	Sodium
Black bean soup,	1.5 cups	174	8	30	2	550
Pitta bread	half	83	3	17	0.4	161
Avocado	¼	82	1	4	8	5
Lettuce, chopped	¼ cup	2	0	0	0	1
Tomato, chopped	half med.	13	0.5	3	0	6
Bean sprouts	¼ cup	2	0.3	0.3	0	0.5
Low fat dressing	2 tbsp.	48	0.5	2	4	236
Apple, medium	one	80	0.3	21	0.5	0
Iced tea	1 cup	2	0	0.5	0	0
Total Lunch		**486**	**13.6**	**77.8**	**14.9**	**959.5**

Dinner

Food Item	Portion	Calories	Protein	Carbs	Fat	Sodium
Pasta noodles, spiral	2 cups	378	13	76	2	3
Pasta sauce	1 cup	170	4	26	8	530
Chicken, white meat	3oz (75g)	162	25	0	6	73
Mixed vegetables	1 cup	107	5	24	0.3	64
French bread	2 pieces	192	6	36	2	426
Tossed mixed salad greens	2 cups	50	2.5	10	0.7	28
Low fat dressing	2 tbsp.	30	2	1	3	368
Water	16oz	0	0	0	0	0
Total Dinner		**1089**	**57.5**	**173**	**22**	**1492**

Snacks

Food Item	Portion	Calories	Protein	Carbs	Fat	Sodium
Yogurt, nonfat, fruit	8oz	115	10	18	0.4	90
Grapes	1 cup	114	1	29	0.9	3
Raisins	50g	145	2.1	69.3	0.4	60
Total Snacks		**374**	**13.1**	**116.3**	**1.7**	**153**
Grand Total		**2429**	**110.1**	**448.7**	**44.1**	**4198.5**

MENU OPTIONS

Having seen the possibilities that are inherent in planning menus which are low in fat, high in carbohydrates, fulfil all your dietary needs and are so low in calories that they will help you lose weight, there is little excuse not to at least attempt to follow a healthy eating plan. Of course there are those who will claim it's all too difficult and there isn't enough variety. Here is a list of low calorie meals that should provide enough variation for even the most jaded palate.

All require little or no cooking skills beyond chopping, boiling, grilling and mixing and so there is no excuse for saying 'it's much too difficult'! Obviously ingredients do vary and the calorie counts are approximate and can be changed instantly if you dollop butter on the baked spud or pour lashings of oil on the salads. For ease of calculation 1oz = 25g.

FIVE BREAKFASTS

1. One 3oz plain bagel, low fat cream cheese, 1 medium banana, black coffee = 410 calories
2. One soft boiled egg, two slices wholewheat toast, low sugar fruit spread (2 tbsp), one cup fresh fruit salad, black coffee = 377 calories
3. 1 cup orange juice, 2oz cereal, 1 cup low fat milk, small banana, black coffee = 500 calories
4. One medium bran muffin, vanilla yogurt = 500 calories
5. 2 slices vegetarian pizza left over from dinner last night! = 500 calories

TEN LUNCHES AND DINNERS

1. **Prawn salad**: 10 steamed or boiled prawns, tossed mixed salad, croutons, roasted red pepper, 7 slices of cucumber, spring onions, low fat dressing, one bread stick and a cup of melon cubes = 395 calories
2. **Turkey sandwich**: 3oz white turkey, mustard, lettuce

leaves, half a tomato inside two wholewheat bread slices, plus an apple = 319 calories

3. **Sports salad**: three cups lettuce, half large tomato, half green pepper, half cup broccoli, half a carrot, one third cup of chick peas, half cup three bean salad, a sprinkling of toasted croutons, 2 tbsp of light dressing = 435 calories

4. **Steak and baked potato**: 3oz (cooked weight) lean-cut flank steak, one medium baked potato, either low fat sour cream or low fat butter substitute, 6 stalks fresh steamed asparagus, plus one cup of strawberries = 390 calories

5. **Grilled salmon**: 3oz grilled salmon steak, one cup long grain brown rice, steamed courgettes, half a tomato, tossed salad leaves, 6 slices cucumber = 484 calories

6. **Chicken and vegetable stir fry**: 3oz chicken breast chopped, 1½ cups oriental vegetables (spring onions, Chinese cabbage, carrots, green beans, mangetout), cup of white rice, plus a cup of strawberries = 503 calories

7. **Pasta with ragu sauce**: 1½ cups pasta (egg-free if possible), ½ cup sauce, one cup steamed string beans, tossed mixed salad low fat dressing = 475 calories

8. **Roast chicken breast and baked potato**: one chicken breast roasted, one medium baked potato, sour cream (non/low fat), cup peas, tossed mixed salad, low fat dressing = 488 calories

9. **Grilled tuna with roasted vegetables**: grilled 3oz tuna steak (or swordfish or any other suitable fish), olive oil for brushing, I cup mixed roasted vegetables (carrots, parsnips, peppers, garlic, courgettes) ½ cup wild rice, 2 cups mixed tossed salad with light dressing, plus kiwi fruit = 502 calories

10. **Grilled mackerel on lentils**: grilled small mackerel, 1½ cups of green lentils with added onion and garlic, 2 cups tossed green salad, plus apple = 500 calories

These are not recipes, just ideas. Here's another. If you look at your list of recommended foodstuffs you should have worked out that beans are good for you. There is nothing wrong with a light lunch of a tin of baked beans (preferably the low sugar ones) on two slices of wholewheat toast. If you are extra hungry you could add a poached egg on top – but not chips – or grill some mushrooms which are high in carbohydrates but low in calories. There may be other flatulent consequences to such a meal but it will still be a low calorie, low fat meal.

There are plenty of vegetarian and low fat recipe books in the shops. The only limit to a healthy diet is your imagination.

ALCOHOL

Well we couldn't go through all these healthy eating suggestions without staggering onto the subject of the demon booze, could we? In Body Food we talked about how alcohol has the frustrating quality of converting itself not into energy but only calories. Most adults have already settled into their own drinking patterns. If you are serious about this exercise programme you will want to cut down your consumption, but at the same time, if you like to have a sociable drink, continue to do so. If you need to have a drink to relax every so often do so, but do be aware of the longterm effects of drinking.

Alcohol has lots of calories and rapidly dissolves any determination that you had to watch what you eat. Alcohol is a depressant and an addictive substance. While drinking over and above one to two glasses of beer or wine a day may produce a feeling of euphoria, it is not an effective weight or stress management technique, nor is it necessary. So think before you drink! Try having a large glass of water in between drinks. It fills you up and slows down the amount of alcohol you consume.

Look at the following chart and see how many pounds you can gain in one year based on what you drink a day:

Alcoholic Drinks

Beverage	Amount (oz)	Calories (one drink)	Weight Gain Per Year with One Drink a Day (lbs)
Regular beer/ale	12	140–50	15
Light beer	12	100	10
Wine, dry table	3.5	87	9
Wine, red table	3.5	74	9
Wine, rose table	3.5	73	8
Wine, white table	3.5	70	7
Wine spritzer	5.0	61	6
Wine, non-alcoholic	3.5	7	1
Gin, rum, vodka, whiskey			
80 proof	1.5	97	10
86 proof	1.5	105	11
90 proof	1.5	110	11
94 proof	1.5	116	12
100 proof	1.5	124	13
Cordials and liqueurs	1.0	100	10
Brandy and cognac	1.0	65	7

Cocktails

Beverage	Amount (oz)	Calories (one drink)	Weight Gain Per Year with One Drink a Day (lbs)
Bloody Mary	5.0	116	12
Daiquiri	2.2	113	12
Frozen Daiquiri	8.0	298	31
Bourbon and soda	8.0	105	11
Gin and tonic	7.5	171	18
Manhattan	2.0	128	13
Margarita	2.7	168	18
Martini	2.5	159	17
Pina Colada	4.7	231	24
Screwdriver	7.0	174	18

That's the bad news. The good news is that you can sip mineral water with a twist of lemon and save all of those calories. If that seems too desolate, try to drink only on the weekends. A person who usually has two glasses of wine per day will lose 12lbs in one year by only having wine on the weekend – or any two days that you choose. Now, how hard can that be . . . and if it is hard, then maybe something else is going on. Walking off alcohol to hasten metabolism is of no help and can be dangerous because muscles can't use alcohol directly, it has to be converted to glucose by the liver. Drinking black coffee will only make you a wide-awake drunk!

QUESTIONS

1. Which of the following is the best bet for giving you the calcium you need? 1oz cheddar cheese, 1 cup broccoli, 1 large egg or 1 cup low-fat milk?

2. Which of the following fats is the most saturated – butter, lard, coconut oil or avocado oil?

3. Which food(s) is/are a good source of beta-carotene, a vitamin A precursor and anti-oxidant – spinach, cantaloupe, carrots, or all of the above?

4. Is vitamin B12 found in meat, poultry and fish, fruits and vegetables or bread, cereal, and rice?

5. Which of these foods has the highest fat content – mayonnaise, sour cream, mustard,or non-dairy creamer?

6. Which foods are highest in potassium – bananas and potatoes, bologna and hot dogs, or rice and oats?

7. Which of the following contains the most cholesterol   whole grains, vegetable oils, fish and poultry or nuts and seeds?

8. Which food group is the highest in the mineral iron – bread and cereal,meat, poultry, fish and beans, fruit and vegetables or grains?

9. Which is highest in Vitamin C – a tomato, an apple, or a pear?

10. Which of the following is a good source of zinc–meat, fish and poultry, whole grains, vegetables or all of the above?

11. Which has more fibre – steak, a glass of milk or an apple?

12. Which of the following is a good source of Vitamin D – oily fish (salmon, tuna, mackerel, and herring), vitamin D fortified milk, sunshine or all of the above

(Answers at the end of the book)

CHAPTER 14

PREPARING FOR BODY HEAT

So you think you're ready. You've been through a lot of training since we started and now you believe you're ready to tackle Body Heat itself. This chapter looks first at what the audition demands and gives some advice on preparing for the bleep test. Then we look in more detail at the demands of each individual test. Andrew Nash gives some personal advice on how to cope with the stresses and strains of both individual events and the competition as a whole. (For more advice on the psychology of competing see Chapter 17: Winning).

Finally we offer a four-week programme geared up to taking part in the auditions for Body Heat. In the following chapters past winners and finalists have generously shared their training schedules and tips with us while Kirstie Chapman gives a personal account of her experiences competing in 1995.

PICKING YOUR PARTNER

Aside from actually going to the auditions, picking the right partner for Body Heat is the most important decision you will make. In the past series of Body Heat partners have been married, engaged or living with each other, or brother and sister but usually they are either friends, friends of friends, colleagues or people who just happen to train in the same gym. There are no hard and fast rules. It is perfectly possible to enter the show with someone who lives on the other side of the country but that might take away much of the enjoyment of the experience.

The first thing to look for is a person whose character and personality either blends with or complements your own. If you have a personality clash and things start to go wrong everything can fall apart. You have to trust that your partner will be giving 110% just as you are. It is also no good if you're a bloke looking for the strongest girl in town if she can't run, or if you're a girl looking for a bloke who can get to Level 17 on the bleep test but has the upper body strength of a butterfly. On very few occasions during the programme has a woman out-performed a man, so don't expect it, but if it happens and it's your partner you have both won a crushing psychological battle over one of the other teams.

'Whatever sex you are, you need to look for strength and character in your partner, the ability to perform when tired, to get good endurance. I wouldn't have entered unless I thought I would stand a good chance of winning,' recalls Andrew Nash. His partner Caroline Rice was married with four children under the age of five – now she has five boys under seven. The very fact that with those domestic arrangements she could maintain such a punishing training schedule shows how dedicated she was. 'She was a very strong lady in mind and body. She had a lot of grit and determination, could handle the pain of working flat out and when you see somebody sweating and drenched and still going for it you know what kind of character they have. She was not scared to work hard and look terrible. She was very strong and powerful, not really a natural runner but so fit she could make it on the bleep test.'

As a partnership you have to be consistent in both training and competition, and supportive and positive in failure. In any long training schedule individuals will have peaks and troughs, and it is up to you to keep your partner motivated through the troughs while they must do the same while for you.

'We have seen that the teams who actually work as a team are the ones that succeed,' says Jeremy Guscott. 'There have been lots of favourites in every heat and the finals, but that has been determined by the one strong partner and what eventually happens is that they don't work well as a team. They just fall short and the team that weren't so good on paper work very hard at helping one another, motivating one another, going through everything together, and they come through to win.'

It is also important to keep things in perspective. Training hard six days a week while holding down a job can quickly equate to 'no life at all'. Make sure you always have one day off and if you spend it with your partner don't talk about training at all. A change can be as good as a rest.

JEREMY'S TRAINING TIP
TRAINING PARTNERS

In Body Heat you have a partner to bounce off which is very important. I used to train a lot with the Bath scrum half Richard Hill who was very disciplined and this summer it is essential for me to get a new training partner. Sally has the luxury of John, her husband, who loves the training, is a big motivator and they work very well together as a team.

So get yourself a training partner, which means you have made a commitment and you don't want to let them down. It is good to have bit of competition – going out against yourself is always difficult because you can ease back, but if you are out there with someone of similar pace and strength you keep going. It is even better if they are faster or stronger than you which gives an easy target to aim for. If you are the stronger one it means you have to work harder to stay that small step ahead.

BODY HEAT: THE AUDITION

The 'bleep test' – formally known as the Multi Stage Fitness test – is designed to test endurance and aerobic fitness and is deeply dreaded by most athletes. Starting off at a slow jog you run a 20m shuttle, turning on the line at the beep, and while the levels get progressively faster you are never sprinting. On the beep test the average 30-year-old male would not reach level 8. Obviously this is a test that requires superb endurance and the best performances will come from middle to long distance runners.

What happens is that the end arrives almost without warning, the line gets further and further away and if you miss three beeps you have to stop. It is not the heart and lungs that give way first, it is the legs – the constant tensing and relaxing of the muscles does drain them. It doesn't matter how fit you are when your legs have gone, in this constant stop, start, turn process sometimes they will not move fast enough for you to get from point a to point b.

You need to practise the bleep test because the turning is very important. It gets easier the more you do it, though it always hurts. If you train for six months at one pace you won't be able to get hold of the bleep test. It is a killer. You can practise doing turns at speed, try to stop and turn and start again when you are tired. Do a really good leg workout, then put yourself through some short shuttle sprints to see how your legs react when they are tired.

At a Body Heat audition a man should be aiming for a minimum of level 13, a woman of level 11. However as the show is looking for all round fitness it is also essential to do well on the press ups.

PRESS UPS

Press Ups have to be carried out according to the prescribed form, with chest brushing the ground to count. As with the bleep test they are done to exhaustion. At a Body Heat audition a man should be aiming for a minimum of 40–50 press ups, a woman a minimum 25–35 press ups.

Eventual selection will depend on both partners being able to fulfil the criteria of both endurance and upper body strength. A man with a bleep test of 17 but only able to do 32 press ups might well fail the audition. You have been warned . . . concentrate on all round fitness.

BODY HEAT: THE SHOW

If you have successfully passed the audition these are the tests you will be expected to go through. Though they are shown in a specific order on television, in fact the shows take place at three different times. So your training schedule should be adjusted accordingly.

THE ENDURANCE EVENT

This takes place on either:

Cycle machine – 4000m
Rowing machine – 2000m
Step machine – 300m (equivalent to 104 floors)
Versa Climba – 400m
Ski machine – 1100m
Schwinn Air – 4000m

The event will last between 6–12 minutes at race pace – which is obviously tougher than training pace. All six competitors in three teams race off together. The winner in each category scores 100, the second 75 points and the third 50.

If you have successfully passed your audition you know what you are going to be doing six weeks in advance, so it is important to make sure that your local gym has that piece of equipment – or something very similar. Familiarize yourself with it, do some distance training on it and then do 1–2 sessions a week at speed. The more you train at that level the more comfortable you will be at it. 'Don't do too many sessions of the race distance itself,' warns Andrew Nash. 'I would do it once a week and do it fresh, come in have a light warm up, stretch and then go straight into it flat out and then call it a day. Don't do it after a hard session because you might get demoralized. Do one final session four days before the competition so you are familiar with the movement. The most difficult are those machines that require more than one movement – the ski machine, the rowing machine, the Versa Climba. Anything that pushes you to the limit is hard but ultimately a race is a race and everyone gets off shattered.'

SPRINT RELAY

This is the first event to be filmed and usually takes place at the National Indoor Arena in Birmingham. It is a 200m sprint relay with the winning team – the first colour to cross the line – scoring 200 points, the second 150 points and the third 100. 'There are tactics involved,' says Andrew Nash. 'It doesn't just have to be girls against girls, boys against boys. Last year, one guy went to race against the girls but it didn't pay off as he didn't get enough lead on the girls for his partner to get home first. The distance may not be far enough for the distance in speed and strength between the sexes to come into play.'

POWER POINT

Body Heat's Strength Test takes place on the Cybex Norm. It is usually measured on the day after the Sprint Relay. The Cybex is an item of physiotherapy equipment and its main component is its central arm. The arm works in a circular direction but when used with different attachments can be used to exercise or test any individual muscle or group of muscles in the body. As a force is applied to the arm it resists, making it harder to move. The more force applied by an individual, the greater the resistance. The arm can be moved with a very light touch, yet the harder you push it, the harder it pushes back.

The rotor has a sensor which measures the force the individual is applying to it at any point during its rotation. This allows a physio to test any muscle or group of muscles across their full range of movement – showing both the weak and strong areas. This gives useful information for training and the management of injuries. For Body Heat they take the information for two muscle actions in both directions, the arm and the leg. Three full movements are made with the leg and three with the arm. The results are averaged and with a simple equation converted to give the average weight moved. But it is not just sheer strength that is measured as a formula gives added points for power. The winner in each category scores 100 points, the second 75 points and the third 50. There are also bonuses of 5 points for combined scores over 230kg for men and 140kg for women. However, you do not know the results of your test until the night of the show.

'The leg movements are quite straightforward,' says Andrew Nash. 'It is like a leg extension and leg curl except it is all one movement. You do three reps on just one leg, you extend and pull back in one movement. The arm movement you cannot train for specifically, you lie on your back with the arm slightly bent and you push down and then pull back. Pushing down you use the chest, the back, the biceps, triceps, forearm and shoulder. It is also the speed of movement as well, not just pure strength, if you are explosively quick out of the blocks. In 1995, Paul Hibbert who was a 400m runner wasn't a massive guy, but he registered higher than someone who was a body-builder, who might have been able to lift more weights but did not register so much explosive strength.'

BODY MATTERS QUIZ

The individuals in the teams take it in turns to sprint to a question point and back. The six questions vary but generally deal with Body Matters – about diet and physiology. The team scores 20 points for each correct answer if you are first back and 10 points if you are right but second or third back. The maximum score for any team is 120 points. 'It may turn out to be crucial at the end,' advises Andrew Nash 'but if you don't do that well, don't get discouraged. You can make the points up on the Batak wall.'

BLEEP TEST

You only have 40 minutes between the Endurance Test and the Bleep Test which isn't much when you have to cool down and warm up again. Mental strength starts to play an important part on the night of the recording in the TV studio. Walking in and out of the studio to discover the results of the Power and Pressure Points can give you an extra mental lift or it can cause a crash. If your team have won the Endurance Test that is 100 points each and you already know the results of the sprint so you could be 200 points up. But a couple of bad results and you're back in second place.

Once again, the winner of the event scores 100 points but in addition there are bonuses of 5 points extra for every two shuttles you complete over level 15 for men and over level 12 for women.

'On the bleep test most people score better on their audition because they haven't already shattered themselves on the endurance test,' says Andrew Nash. 'Guys doing 17:3 in audition might only make 16:3 on the day. You have to decide at the end of day whether it is worth knackering yourself on that event for the sake of 10 or 20 points when one hit on the Tri Batak wall is worth 10 points.'

PRESSURE POINTS

Body Heat pressure points cannot be trained for specifically as they are designed to test how well the competitors react under stress. For one programme in the 1995 series competitors had to travel up to the Lake District. The male team member had to abseil down from Devil's Bridge, collect a buoy from the river's surface, climb back up, with assistance from the female member of the team, hand the buoy over and the girl had to sprint 200m to the finish line. Now, that sounds easy enough except that dangling inches above a fast flowing stream three of the four men managed to clip their carabina onto the safety rope. This meant that they had to haul themselves up by sheer upper body strength wasting valuable seconds on the way. Everything had gone fine in practice but in the white hot heat of competition brains can fuse.

Other pressure points vary widely. The 'Biathlon' involves running off a 100ft cliff on a zip rope line, picking up an ammunition box and charging up the side of densely wooded hill to a target point, where one competitor has to hit three targets with an air rifle. Then it's up to the next target point where the other competitor has to repeat the process, then up to the top of the hill. That is a test that requires both stamina and the ability to concentrate the mind on holding the body steady. Other Pressure Points can include an 'Aerial Assault Course' which involves swinging Tarzan-like through the trees, then wading out to a speedboat and driving as fast as possible through a slalom course; or erecting a giant Body Heat banner below an 80ft suspension bridge. 'Castle Assault' involves canoeing across a lake in a Canadian open canoe and ascending a 70ft tower. 'The Navy Log Run' demands competitors carry a log through a Navy assault course, then attach it to the back of a quad bike and drive 40m to the finish. In 'Waterfalls' the teams have to negotiate a section of the Royal Navy's waterfall assault course in the Brecon Beacons.

As you can see, each Pressure Point is very different. But what they have in common is to demand that the competitors are not afraid to get down and get dirty. And that they work as a team. If you suffer from a fear of heights, as people have in the past, that is bad luck but most people can conquer their fear, perhaps only temporarily, if they are motivated enough. Sheer brute force is not enough, Pressure Point winners have learnt to think on their trainers.

The closest one gets to preparing for Pressure Points is to either join the Territorial Army or go on an Adventure Training weekend. But to do that – and it could be fun – will require taking time off training. If there is time it's worth learning to handle a climbing rope which will enable you to discover any residual fear of heights, how to abseil and most important of all it will help with upper body strength. Climbing ropes, though an essential part of military training, are not available in most gyms because of the specialized techniques and the height of ceiling required.

The winning team scores 200 points, the second 150 points and the third 100.

TRI BATAK

You have perhaps another 30 minutes to recover after the bleep test. 'Everyone is shattered now,' says Andrew Nash. 'It's the last event and you want to get it over with, put everything into that last burst.'

Tri Batak is four minutes of really hard work, with both partners working hard in tandem. The machines are rigged up so that both partners contribute to the same result. Between you, you have to cover 200m on a swim bench, 400m on a cycle and 800m on the running machine. The machines are rigged so you can only finish together and when the monitor has counted down to zero you get off and onto the next one. When the running has finished you get off and start on the Batak wall, alternately hitting a target. It has to be hit firmly or it does not register.

The swim bench involves an arm movement. Some people just punch their arms forward and pull back, others do a real freestyle/ front crawl technique to get more distance. The idea is to keep the flywheel inside the machine moving to cover both speed and distance. You should come off with maybe a minute to go and, with each hitting out alternately on the Batak wall to get 10 points a target, you should be able to get 500 points. However the bats are quite small and it is possible to mis-hit them, lunge for one target, come back and not r-ealize you haven't hit it correctly.

'There are people who are so exhausted by this point,' says Andrew Nash, 'that they have lost their coordination – or perhaps they simply aren't coordinated in the first place. You are better taking your time making sure you hit the middle of the target, looking straight ahead, and not to the side to see how the others are doing. It's all about focus. You can hear the noise from your partner hitting, you can feel it and so you lunge forward again.'

'In the first year when I competed, one of the guys was a national triathlete and they were way ahead until the Batak wall where they blew it. They stopped before they had to. It is important to be aware of this in the last few weeks of training because you can lose so many points through not having good reflexes. It is about speed on the feet, reaction time, and having your brain still working even though your body wants to collapse.'

WINNERS

It is not always the very fittest who triumph in Body Heat. Mental strength is important, but winning your heat is not enough. There are six heats and only three finalists. So you have to push yourself and each other that extra metre to make the final . . . which is another ball game altogether.

THE GRAND FINAL

Getting to the final is a massive achievement of which 99% of the population of Great Britain are incapable. Winning the final – becoming Body Heat Champions – is another matter.

For a start there is scarcely a break between the heats, getting on a plane to America or South Africa, or wherever the programme makers have planned for the future. Then you have a week to get over jet lag, scope out and maybe psych out the opposition and compete in a series of different events. These all take place outside so the environment plays a vital part. Anyone whose training has been inside the gym is at an immediate disadvantage. The events, too, are often more adventure training/ fitness in their concept, so that the ability to think fast while tired is essential.

In the first series Andrew Nash and his partner Caroline Rice came second to Debbie Moulton and Jeremy Tiffen. In the second series Kirstie Chapman and Andy McKee lost to Cindy Parsons and Simon Amery. Both times it all came down to the last event – a mountain bike race. 'Caroline was incredibly strong,' recalls Andrew Nash, 'but she hadn't ridden a mountain bike until five days before the event. To have to tackle that, learn to use 20 gears when you are shattered from earlier events simply proved too much. She started off in too low a gear and her legs could not make it.' A year later Kirstie began her race in too low a gear, losing ground she could never make up. Riding bikes in the gym is easy, they don't go anywhere.

'That proves that you don't always want to do your training within the confines of the gym, so do it outside to get a feel for the natural environment,' says Andrew Nash. 'It is not the same as being on a stationary cycle or a rowing machine. There is the feeling and coordination on water or a mountain path. In the final you need to have a bit of luck but it is mainly in the head where a good couple will come through. You have to have a consistent partner, one who while they might not win every- thing will come second in everything, you cannot afford to come bottom in any event.'

A Four Week Programme leading up to an audition for Body Heat

Commitment = Five times a week. Three sessions in the gym, never on consecutive days. Two other sessions, one running, one other personal choice. Make sure you have at least one day of total rest when you take no exercise at all

Gym Programme:
Warm up and full body stretches
Light jog or cycle 6–10 minutes
Aerobic Machines:
Three: two steady ones and one fast one for intensity

Cycle	= 8–12 minutes
	Race mode / random programme
	80–100 rpm, Gear/levels 5–12
Step	= 8–12 minutes / 100–150 floors
	Manual programme = level 8–10
	Climbing action
Rowing Machine	= 6–12 minutes
	Programme 2 = 3,000–6,000m
	Level 15 – 36–45 strokes per minute
Run	= 10–15 minutes
	Manual = 0% incline (flat)
	Run at 6mph, 7mph, 8mph, 9mph, 10mph, 11mph. Every minute take the speed up 1mph. This will mimic the bleep test in that the machine is going faster and faster as the bleeps get quicker and quicker.

Hill Sprints (once a week)
8–10 × 50m
Recovery jog down (30 seconds max)
(see Chapter 11: Running for further information on Hill Sprints)
Weight Machines:
Resistance Machines: Six

Body Part	Machine	Reps	Sets	Weight
Upper Body	Bench Press	8–12	3	Medium
Shoulders	Shoulder Press	8–12	3	Medium
Back	Lateral Pull down	8–12	3	Medium
or	Pull Ups	8–12	3	Medium
Triceps	Tricep Dips	8–12	3	Medium
Quads	Leg Extension	8–12	3	Medium
Hamstrings	Leg Curls	8–12	3	Medium

EXTRAS

PRESS UPS

In order to pass the audition you will need to be able to do a lot of press ups. You should have been practising them in your personal circuit for some weeks but it never hurts to practise getting into the routine.

Try to do at least 3 sets of 30–50 press ups (1–2 minutes rest between sets) at least three times a week.

You should be running twice a week in addition to the gym programme, so do the press up sets in conjunction with the runs/hills sessions, either at the end (take a five-minute rest period while you stretch and cool down from the run) or the beginning after the stretch.

ROPE CLIMBING

Climbing ropes is a great exercise for upper body strength. While it uses the same muscles as pull ups, the thrill generated by being 20ft up in the air adds a certain frisson and adrenalin rush. It can be difficult to find gyms with ropes outside of the services and climbing centres, but if you can, do. Get some lessons in basic climbing technique and practise going up and down a 20ft rope as many times as you can.

The other reason is to give you a possible edge in a Body Heat Pressure Point. In the past three series a high proportion of the Pressure Points have involved abseiling or rope climbing in some way. If you are at least familiar with the techniques it might give you that vital edge. It is also very important to practise with your partner. If one of you suffers from vertigo, it's better to find out now than when everything depends on scaling a castle wall.

SPRINT SESSIONS

Do a couple of 200m sprint sessions to hone your speed. Go to your local athletics training track to get used to the feel of running on a track, the way your body feels going round the bends. Do 5x200m sprints with a 200m jog for recovery.

PLYOMETRIC SESSIONS

Once a week maximum. Plyometrics is an extremely good method for adding explosive power to your fitness. However, if you want to incorporate plyometrics into your training routine always do it with at least one other person and make sure that the initial sessions are conducted under the supervision of someone who knows what they are doing. See Chapter 10: Turning Up The Heat for more details on Plyometrics.

Remember, Body Heat is a television programme – they want people who are super fit, who look good but who are also enjoying themselves so . . .

PRACTISE SMILING AND LAUGHING!!!

JEREMY'S TRAINING TIP

COMPETING IN GENERAL

There is always a first time for competition and it can be daunting. In the early days I would have a horrible sickly feeling in the pit of my stomach that just would not go away and I'd feel I was going to be sick – some players I know actually vomit through nerves. I still notice the spectators when I first go out, it's an almighty rush of noise that hits you and you can't help but be aware of it. But when the whistle goes it is like a switch being pulled. They disappear and I just follow the ball.

Most people thrive on adrenalin and the fear of going into the unknown – that is what keeps me going. I love playing rugby because I really don't know what is going to happen when I get out on the pitch, but there are some who fall short perhaps because they get distracted by the crowd or simply overburdened by their own expectations. It is hard to do initially but keep focused on your goal and other distractions will vanish.

COMPETING IN BODY HEAT

Body Heat competitors are very intense people who are there to do very well. They want to win and they have nothing else on their minds. However, often competitors really don't know what to expect when they get in the studio, it is very upbeat, everybody has their supporters and the adrenalin is pumping.

They get tighter and tighter as the day goes on. They come with great big smiles and a bit of kidology going on with other teams, but once they get into Lycra on the studio floor they are ready to go and they are on their own. Some respond very well, others, through no fault of their own, maybe timing, maybe nerves, fall a little bit short.

The biggest fear that any competitor has is that it is harder than they expected and they really can't perform up to their expectations. In Body Heat it is so important that if you have under-performed there is a partner who can pick you up and say you can do better next time. One thing everybody can take away with them is that they came, they tried, they never gave up and they can take great pride in that.

CHAPTER 15

COMPETING IN BODY HEAT

Kirstie Chapman, 24, is the manager of the Fitness Exchange in Fenchurch Street, London. In January 1995 her then boss Andy McKee came to her with an offer she couldn't refuse. This is her account of the next three months, when she and Andy strove to become the Body Heat Champions, of the sacrifices it entailed and what it is like to compete . . . and perhaps even to win.

It all began one day back in early January. Following three weeks of intense drinking and serious eating over the Christmas break something drastic had to be done to get back into the world of fitness. I was just about to go out on my first run of 1995 when Andy came running over, smiling from ear to ear with a large Body Heat poster in his hand. 'You'll do it,' he said in a sadistic tone of voice. 'Do what?' I replied, rather hesitantly.

He then went on to explain about the TV programme which involved couples competing in various tortuous gym challenges. We signed up for the auditions which involved the infamous bleep test. However we were confident of being one of the 24 couples chosen, despite approximately 2,000 couples taking part overall. When the all important phone call came through the adrenaline started pumping and our excitement levels hit the roof – yes, we were in!

There was, however, a part of me that had already begun to visualize the hundreds of killer training sessions that lay ahead – was I really wise to go ahead with it? I soon convinced myself that it was going to be a fun and enjoyable experience! Before

191

the serious training started, I don't think I fully appreciated the meaning of the phrase 'an intense training session'. Many sessions drove me close to tears – the pain, the agony, the constant pressure of the whole thing really got to me at times.

Being more of a beer-drinking, pub-going person than Andy, I especially found the weekend training a lot harder than he did. Every Saturday or Sunday we either went to the gym, to the track, or out for a run. The hardest thing for me was that I couldn't even go out that night, order a pint (or 10) saying 'Well at least I've earned this!' From the beginning of February to the end of March the training got progressively harder, longer, faster and more intense. I would look back at a session we did two weeks earlier and it would look relatively easy. I think my rate of improvement was faster than Andy's, simply because I had a lot further to go until I reached my peak – Andy was already halfway up his hill at the beginning! Having said this, the training Andy was doing before was totally different in nature. Converting from winter training for the 800m to training for a broad range of events requiring speed, stamina and strength was hard in itself. I know Andy found each and every session very tough and even he got a lot fitter (which I didn't think was possible).

Our first filming took place in Birmingham in March and we travelled up there on a coach with the production crew and our fellow competitors. Despite our preconceived ideas about the nature of the competitors all our fellow athletes were extremely friendly and it was good to meet so many like-minded souls. We made quite a few friends from the series and still keep in touch with them.

We all arrived at the hotel and first thing on the agenda was to collect the dreaded Lycra! We were given all our kit in a Body Heat bag, then scurried back to our rooms to try on the skimpy luminous outfits. The next thing all the competitors were out in the corridors laughing hysterically at each other – there was a mass of pink, red, blue, green and yellow. Each show had three couples and we had drawn the short straw – red and pink. The thought of appearing in front of 10 million people kitted out like a pink bunny nearly made me pack my bags and head straight home. However a few kind souls told me it wasn't too bad, which I was just about falling for when suddenly Andy came out with 'Don't be fooled by that lot – you look awful!' I told him he didn't look too hot himself! Then it was off to the National Indoor Arena for our briefing on the next day's events.

During the international athletics meeting on the Saturday we were taken down to the warm up area where we prepared ourselves for races alongside the likes of Linford Christie, John Regis and Frankie Fredericks (not that I'm a name dropper or anything). Then it was the real thing – our first event of the competition, a 2 × 200m sprint relay. We watched the other competitors impatiently and nervously, then it was our turn. We were amazed at the number of spectators watching us and, as we approached the arena we were hit by a cauldron of sound. We had a close heat, the closest of the series actually, but fortunately we won, thanks, I think to Andy's experience of track running and tactics. The crowd seemed to enjoy the exciting finish and we got a great ovation on our lap of honour. The first event was in the bag.

For one couple who were originally going to be on our show it proved to be their last event. During the race the man pulled a hamstring and they were forced to withdraw – all of that hard work for nothing.

On the Sunday we were taken to Manchester United's training ground and were surprised to see how unglamorous it was, considering they are one of the best football clubs in the world. Inside we had a look at the piece of equipment we were going to be tested on – the Cybex 6000 – a strange contraption which required an arm movement that was very hard to simulate in the gym. To film each of the 48 competitors it took over 15 hours, a very long and tedious day. Even at the end of it we weren't told any results. They were to be announced on the studio night which was a few weeks away.

After this weekend it was back to hard graft in the gym.

We altered our training slightly and concentrated more on endurance, interspersed with some quality track sessions. Andy convinced me to join his athletic club and train with them on Tuesday evenings. A few wintry Tuesdays later I began to question myself, 'How on earth did Andy ever get me to agree to this one?' I thought it must have been discussed one drunken evening, but then I remembered I hadn't been on a serious session for a while. It was then it really hit me. I had said 'no' to many social get-togethers and 'yes' to all sorts of bizarre training sessions – what was happening to me? A visit to the local GP soon put my mind at rest. He put it down to a rare condition known as McKee-itis, a condition whereby one's brain becomes totally obsessed with training and sport.

I was a touch concerned at first but then was comforted by the knowledge that the disease wasn't permanent and that the symptoms were reversible. Back in the gym our training turned very specific with some rather imaginative inventions for simulating the Batak wall that required boxing gloves and two pairs of extremely tired legs. Again, each session pushed us both to the limit and a new higher level of fitness was accomplished every day.

Our Pressure Point was filmed up in the Lake District and involved Andy abseiling off Devil's Bridge into a river, collecting a buoy, then a joint effort to pull him back up onto the bridge. Then I had to sprint 200m to set off a flare. The actual abseil went very smoothly but it all went wrong on the climb back as Andy clipped onto the wrong rope by mistake. However, 3 out of 4 couples made the same mistake, so fortunately we escaped with a lucky second place.

Our next – and biggest – challenge was the main studio night. This was the one we were really looking forward to and put lots of training into. We arrived at the Carlton TV studio in Nottingham at midday and spent all afternoon being given the run down on the night's events. We began to get nervous and it soon got to the stage when we just wanted to get started. Eventually the recording of the show got under way.

The first event we both won easily, two first places on the

bike race with plenty to spare. One other girl went off really fast and I kept up with her but she blew out and I kept going. I could see how the other two were doing on the screen on my bike so I slowed up towards the end. There weren't any bonus points at stake so I didn't want to end up knackering myself early on. Next was the quiz. In the practice that afternoon both Andy and I had done really well and had answered everything correctly, but on the actual night it all went horribly wrong. Our excuse is . . . erm . . . being a health club manager and assistant manager the pressure to perform well on this was so intense it got to us a bit. Under normal circumstances we'd have done much better (I hope you've fallen for that one).

To make up for this disappointment we were informed we had both won the strength test at Manchester United. I think 'over the moon' and 'gob-smacked' were the appropriate expressions.

The dreaded bleep test was next, an event that Andy and I were both fairly confident about. We were pleased with our performance and both picked up bonus points. Andy got the highest score of the whole series and I was the second highest We were delighted but pretty tired. The bleep test is really the ultimate fitness challenge and the better you are the harder it is. The production crew told us that we were on course for a place in the final but to guarantee it we had to go like lightning in the mini-triathlon. That went smoothly and so we scored well in the Batak (thanks mainly to our makeshift Batak simulator in the gym). Our total score was 1,570, giving us a comfortable win on the show but also giving us second place on the leaders board. However there were still two more shows to go, so our seats on that plane to Atlanta weren't 100% guaranteed.

We had to wait two full days to hear. On the last night Andy was at a party and received about 11 phone calls from Carlton TV telling him the latest on that night's show. It wasn't until midnight that it was confirmed. We'd made it to the grand final in Atlanta. The main thing now was to get some sleep as the next day we had to be at Gatwick ready to go. Our Lycra and passports were packed and before we knew it we were airborne. Although there were only six competitors on board, 44 other seats were taken up with production crew – producers, directors, camera crew, doctors, physios, Sally Gunnell, Mike Smith and Jeremy Guscott.

On arrival in Atlanta we were greeted with a scorching hot summer's day and were briefed on the week's challenges and events. Following indirect questioning and friendly chit chat all the competitors had each other's strengths and weaknesses sussed. The competition was certainly going to be close. As some events only took a few hours to film we had quite a lot of free time and we certainly made the most of it.

The first event was the 3000m running race which went fairly well with a first place for Andy and a second for myself. I was quite disappointed as I led all the way and got pipped on the line by the blue team's Cindy. It was a tough uphill course through a national park at the foot of Stone Mountain. Unfortunately it was quite hard to appreciate the view at the time. The next two events took place at a high school and involved baseball and American Football.

In the baseball event we had to sprint around the diamond and pass each other the ball – well that was what we were meant to do. Disaster struck and we dropped the ball. For this we came last and we were furious. As we went off on our own for a sulk we didn't realize just how costly that drop would prove. We redeemed ourselves in the American Football with a tie for first place. I was delighted as this put us back in contention. Andy was just relieved to get through with his suspect shoulders in one piece. He dislocated his left shoulder years ago playing rugby and raising it over his shoulder can cause it to pop out.

Two days later came the fourth event. Unless you saw the show you probably won't believe that we flew a plane, but fly a plane we did. Overcoming air sickness was uppermost in the contestants' minds; landing the plane with one's lunch safely digesting was far more important than points. Fortunately Andy and I were the only ones to succeed here. It was an amazing experience and incredibly exciting. We were challenged with shooting down (by laser) a target plane in as quick a time as possible. Our combined time was an agonizing two seconds slower than the yellow team, so we just missed out on first place.

It was all square going into the last day – anyone could win. The morning's event was white water rafting, fantastically exciting but not a true test of fitness, though it was pretty tough on the arms. Again we missed out on first place being only three seconds behind the blue team. Overall with just the cycle event to go the yellows couldn't win. All I had to do was beat Cindy and Andy had to beat Simon of the blues and the luxury trip around the world was ours – along with the title of 1995 Body Heat Champions. Andy was convinced we could win and was all fired up and ready to go.

The cycle was a tough climb of about a mile up a mountain on mountain bikes. As the race began I had a problem with my gears and ended up chasing the rest of the competitors. It was both a physical and a mental struggle. Soon Andy and Simon were out of sight. All I could see was Cindy, Sarah and Paul with Cindy way up front. Just to catch up a few metres I'd lost at the beginning was next to impossible, the hill was too steep. When I finally got to the top I knew we hadn't won.

All I wanted to know was where did Andy come. I threw my bike down, hobbled over to him. 'Did you win?' I inquired. 'Yes,' he replied. My heart sank. I felt so guilty. I'd let him down in a big way. Ten pints later that night things didn't seem quite so depressing. Somehow I managed to pull myself together and join in celebrating the end of one of the most unforgettable weeks in my life. At the end of the day it was taking part, not winning, that mattered – though winning would have been a nice bonus.

On our return I went straight out and bought myself a mountain bike with some of the prize money. I cycle to work every day and am now very competent at changing gears!!

CHAPTER 16

ALTERNATIVE TRAINING SCHEDULES

To become a Body Heat competitor you do not have to be a full-time fitness professional – but you do have to be fanatical. If you have reached the stage at which you can even consider trying out for the programme you are already extremely fit. To actually win requires a little extra something.

To give you an idea of the intensity of the training schedules we have spoken to competition winners and heat victors from the past series of Body Heat. What you will be able to see from these training schedules is the variety of exercise you can take to achieve the desired result. What there is no getting away from is the intensity of the training.

Cindy Parsons and Simon Amery were the second Body Heat winners in 1995. Cindy works in a fitness centre while Simon is a policeman. Cindy has given us her training schedule in the weeks before she competed. It is a gruelling, unforgiving schedule. But since she won neither Cindy nor Simon have slowed down much – as their current training schedules demonstrate. Similarly Jeremy Tiffen who won in 1994 maintains his fitness to play rugby. It doesn't get any easier the fitter you become.

'As you can see,' says Cindy, 'it is more or less a cross-training programme. Both Simon and I were strong in all the areas that go to make up physical fitness – speed, endurance and strength – and we had to work on increasing our abilities in all areas. It is no good being a good long distance runner, because they are usually not good cyclists or very strong because they have no need to be.'

'None of the training sessions was easy. I believe in pushing yourself very hard in every session, by doing that you get much more benefit. When it comes down to competition you know how good you are.'

CINDY'S WEEKLY TRAINING SCHEDULE IN 1995 (UP TO AND INCLUDING COMPETITION)

MONDAY

Running – 2–3 miles at 6.5–7 mins per mile pace
Versa Climber – 10 mins
Gym – Back/chest/abs /legs

TUESDAY

Versa Climber – 2 × 10 mins sessions with a 5 mins rest period in the middle
Turbo Trainer (cycling) – 30 mins hard and fast
Gym – Deltoids/arms/abs/legs

WEDNESDAY

Running – 2 miles in 13 mins 43 secs
Circuit Training – 30 secs on, 15 secs off ×30 through various exercises – Squat Thrusts, Press Ups always following arms, leg, trunk rotation
Skipping – 1 min on, 15 secs off ×10, as fast as I could
Ghosting – 30 secs on/15 secs off ×20. This is a squash player's exercise using a court but no ball; it's good for honing speed and fast recovery times

THURSDAY

Gym – Back/chest/abs/legs
NO AEROBIC EXERCISE TODAY

FRIDAY

Turbo Trainer (cycling) – 30 mins hard
Versa Climber – 2 × 10 mins sessions with a 5 mins rest period
in the middle

SATURDAY

Gym – Deltoids/arms/abs/legs

SUNDAY

DAY OFF !!!

Gym session

Gym sessions varied every two sessions. Monday and Tuesday I
concentrated on muscular endurance, Thursday and Friday
were for muscular strength.

Monday: deltoids/arms/abs/legs. 20 reps on each exercise
machine, doing each one 3 times in rotation.
Tuesday: back/chest/abs/legs. 20 reps on each exercise
machine, doing each one 3 times in rotation.
Thursday: back/chest/abs/ legs. I would do five sets of reps on
each machine, increasing the weight raised as I lowered the reps. The first set was 15, the second 12,
then 8, 6 and 6.
Friday: Deltoids/arms/abs/legs. I would do five sets of reps
on each machine, increasing the weight raised as
I lowered the reps. The first set was 15, the second
12, then 8, 6 and 6.

Running

I would always run for 2–3 miles, at the 6.5–7 mins mile pace,
sometimes a bit quicker depending on how tired my legs were.
As part of the Body Heat competition we had to do a 2 × 200m

races. As I am fast anyway I didn't really have to train for this specifically. Simon and I went to a track once before the race just to sharpen up.

Circuit training

This was viewed as an anaerobic workout, concentrating on explosive movements hence good for recovery.

Versa climber

This was our Endurance race on the show so we were looking to go as fast as we possibly could for a maximum of 10 mins. It actually lasted for about 7 mins which was a relief as the Climber is an extremely hard piece of equipment.

Turbo trainer

I would always spend 30 mins on my turbo trainer cycle as it increases endurance. I would vary RPMS and gears at every session.

Skipping and ghosting

Ghosting is more anaerobic than skipping but both are very good for aiding recovery time and increasing leg strength. Skipping when tired also helps sharpen up your mental faculties and coordination. If you get it wrong you can trip over the rope.

Other equipment

Most weeks I varied what I did so I didn't get too bored. Boredom is the biggest danger in training, if you lose that mental edge, you lose the will to win. These are various extras I would do in place of – or in addition to – the usual routine:

> L-Step Machine – 15/30 mins hard or fast at level 11/12
> L-Cycle – 15/30 mins at level 7/8
> Rowing – 15/30 mins at number 7

'I would say that I am fitter now than during the filming of Body Heat,' warns Cindy. 'I currently do 1½–2 hours training per day. I am still working around the same pieces of equipment – Turbo, One-Step, Rower, Running etc. Now I am lifting much heavier weights so I am bigger and stronger. I am also running faster. I do believe running is the best form of exercise – it is just so hard. I always feel the most tired after a run.'

CINDY'S CURRENT TRAINING SCHEDULE (1996)

MONDAY

Running – 2–3 miles
Gym – back/chest/abs

TUESDAY

Gym – deltoids/arms/abs
Ghosting and skipping
Turbo Trainer (cycling) – 30 mins hard and fast

WEDNESDAY

Gym – legs only
Running – 2–3 miles
L-Step – 30 mins hard and fast

THURSDAY

Gym – back/chest/abs

FRIDAY

Gym – Deltoids/armsabs
Running – 2–3 miles
L-Step – 15 mins hard and fast
Rowing – 15 mins

SATURDAY

Gym – legs
Turbo Trainer (cycling) – 30 mins hard

SUNDAY

DAY OFF !!!

'I am looking forward to the Champion of Champions show next year' warns Cindy. 'As I am fitter the competition had better watch out.'

SIMON AMERY'S CURRENT WEEKLY TRAINING SCHEDULE

Simon Amery's schedule is very different from Cindy's in that the majority of his aerobic exercise comes from playing squash three times a week. Squash is a superb form of aerobic exercise in that it demands both explosive speed, fast recovery times and, ultimately, endurance. Andrew Nash spent a lot of time playing badminton to speed his reflexes, demanding as it does sharp turns, endurance and explosive power. Squash is good for heart and lungs but it is not a game for people who are unfit to begin with. At the level at which Simon plays it is worth remembering the old adage, 'You do not play squash to get fit, you get fit to play squash'.

He also stretches for at least 10 minutes on each gym session and warms up properly before a squash game. Gym sessions consist of a flat out 20-minute workout on a different piece of exercise equipment each time – to add variety – followed by strength/endurance exercises targeting different muscular groups.

MONDAY

10 mins stretching
5 kilometre run on treadmill in 17 mins 45 seconds or less
Leg Press – medium weight, 25, 20, 15 reps
Leg Extension – medium weight, 25, 20, 15 reps
Lunges – 30kg 3 × 30 reps
Stomach Crunches – 3 × 50 reps
Waist Crunches – 3 × 50 reps

TUESDAY

10 mins stretching
20 mins on stationary bike – flat out
Chest Press – medium weight 20, 15, 12 reps
Dumbbell Flies – 15kg dumbbell 20, 15, 12 reps
Pec Deck – 45kg 15, 12, 10 reps

WEDNESDAY

Squash – 1 hour hard aerobic workout

THURSDAY

Squash – 1 hour hard aerobic workout

FRIDAY

10 mins stretching
L-Step – 20 mins flat out
Pull Ups – 12, 10, 10 reps
Lateral Pull Downs – 50kg 20, 20, 15 reps
Front Pull Downs – 50kg 20, 20, 15 reps
Alternate Bicep Curls 15kg 25, 20, 20 reps
Barbell Curls – 30kg 20, 15, 12 reps

SATURDAY

Squash – 45 mins to 1 hour hard aerobic workout

SUNDAY

DAY OFF !!!

JEREMY TIFFEN'S TRAINING TIPS

Jeremy Tiffen and Debbie Moulton won the first Body Heat competition in 1994. Jeremy, 25, is a student teacher who also works as a fitness instructor. 'I had met Debbie at a staff party,' he recalls, ' and we decided to enter the competition. I had no idea how big it was and only entered because I lived close to where some of the auditions were being held. After looking at the events I designed a fitness routine myself.'

Jeremy's prime sport is rugby union which gives the lie to those who claim rugger players aren't very fit! He is a scrum half who has played in the Courage League Third Division for Richmond and Moseley. 'At the first training and fitness session at the beginning of the season I always expect to come in the top three,' he says, ' especially on the bleep test.' On Body Heat

Jeremy certainly proved he is immensely strong, coming out top on the Cybex machines.

His current winter training schedule revolves around rugby. There are two weekly club training sessions of 90 minutes which concentrate on a mixture of skill, tactical training and endurance followed by an 80-minute game on Saturdays. 'We do a lot of anaerobic work, high intensity exercises with little recovery time, plyometric exercises, sprint drills and contact work,' he explains. 'In addition I always do two 40-minute runs a week on the treadmill covering a minimum of 6 miles always making sure that my body is working at 70% of its MHR and 2 weight-training sessions of an a hour each. At my weight-training sessions I am concentrating on strength for rugby, so by reducing the weight on the different machines and increasing the number of reps I do, I get higher muscular endurance. For strength, I increase the weights and do less reps.'

CHAPTER 17

WINNING

What is it that drives sportsmen and women on? Why do they put themselves through training and exercise schedules that make ordinary mortals pale at the reading? They give up a normal social life, a family life, perhaps even a love life; they watch their diet fanatically, they seldom drink and even then it's always with one eye on the calorie counter and the hangover clock. They are out on the track come rain come shine, come blizzard come heat wave. They push themselves to the very edge and beyond what the human body is capable of. But why?

Because they want to win.

Picture Sally Gunnell before her 400m hurdles final in Barcelona. Standing there one of the eight best in the world – all eight trained up into peak form, their whole year, perhaps their whole life geared up to the next 53 seconds. At that level only one of them can win and that will be the one who wants it most, whose desire is greatest.

Jeremy Guscott and Sally Gunnell are both at the very top of their chosen sports, but there were times in their careers when they came across people who beat them, who were better than them, whose birthright included more fast twitch muscles or greater lung capacity. But for various reasons those people stopped competing or got injured and couldn't face the long haul back to fitness or their desire to win faded. In 1993–94 Jeremy had a deep-seated groin injury that he could not seem to shake off. It was threatening his career, and the only thing to do was to let nature take its course and then get really fit again.

'You only reach a peak by training ever so hard and getting in the matches and then staying injury-free,' he says. 'There have been times in the past when I know I've reached a level of fitness which it is physically impossible to go beyond unless I have blood transfusions, injections all that sort of stuff. But I can't stop. If I ever drop down from training I do lose my edge. If I lose my edge I stop winning. At the highest level it is all about winning. People talk about entertainment, about being nice, being a sportsman – but all those are secondary to the goal of winning. To being the best.'

In Body Heat every competitor is fighting three simultaneous battles. One is internal, against yourself, fighting every step, every push of the way to make your body go faster, go further and for longer. The second is individual, against your two opponents – you have to make sure that you cross the finishing line before they do to get maximum points. The third is a team battle because you have to physically and mentally support your partner. To win Body Heat you have to win all three battles, but first you have to learn to win each type of battle.

When he was serving in the Royal Marines, Andrew Nash was in the British squad for the biathlon, a combination of cross country skiing and rifle shooting, competing against nations – the Norwegians, the Russians, the East Germans – where skiing is a way of life. 'It is the hardest sport you will ever do,' he says. 'You are using not only your arms and legs but your back. It's like a Marathon on skis, you carry a rifle on your back, and halfway through the race you have to stop and shoot at targets. The fitter you were the quicker your pulse came down for the shooting to be accurate. On a 20km race where you stop four times and shoot each time, if you miss a target you get a one-minute penalty added to your time. On the 10km race where you stop twice, you have to do penalty loops of a 200m track. The Norwegians didn't have a good reputation for shooting so they skied faster to make up for it.

'Each time I went into a race I set myself a realistic goal, demanding my body make an improvement each time, to cut a minute off my time and to make sure that my heart rate was not racing so fast that the rifle jumped and I missed some of the targets. I love the thrill of competing, and the desire to win drives me on. It's not the same for everybody. It is not enough to compete against yourself.

'In my opinion, competition is something you either thrive on or die on. People can rise to the occasion or, as they say, totally lose the plot. With some people, their adrenalin is pumped up so high before the competition begins that it drowns them, they drain themselves and lose their strength. A lot of people freeze – especially those not used to competing – so training should not just include competing against yourself but against other people too.'

Many gyms have introduced internal promotions to encourage competition. Or you can make sure that you do a lot of your training with a mate of equal or greater ability to yourself. Go onto Step Machines next to each other, set yourself 100 floors or a time of seven and half minutes, and then see who is the first one to finish. At the same time as you are going for victory you will learn to keep an eye on what your mate is doing, so you are aware of what is going on around you that can spur you on to greater exertions .

Such training helps instil a mental strength, a confidence in your own abilities that is essential in endurance events. Before Andrew Nash did his Endurance race, Olympic gold medalist Chris Boardman showed how fast he could be. Andrew was faster. 'I was fortunate enough to beat his time,' says Andrew. 'I didn't intend to do that but I knew I could take it fairly fast and keep it there, whereas those who don't compete on regular basis don't know how their bodies are going to react to going fast straightaway. A regular competitor will always have an advantage. That I beat Chris Boardman's time on the cycle was irrelevant, compared to the fact that I was crossing the line first. That was all that was on my mind and all that mattered. No one remembers second place.'

Winning comes from mental strength. If your programme lacks variety your mind will become stale and it might take a split second longer to shift up that extra gear. Throughout the programme we have stressed the need for variety, so if you're feeling jaded, inject a change, a game of five-a-side football or volleyball – anything that involves other people. Aerobics and step aerobics classes are a very good way of countering boredom if you're not getting the same kind of buzz from the type of exercise you are doing, if you feel you need a bit of a challenge, that your coordination isn't very good, or if you just want to go with your friends.

Try to get used to the adrenalin buzz that comes with performing in front of an audience. Pre-competition routines should always be simple and natural. If you are competing regularly always use the same warm-up procedures/routines and eat the same pre-match meal. All of this will help you keep focused on the task ahead. At the same time don't overtrain or over-compete. Sally Gunnell does not race every week of the year. She deliberately focuses on a small number of races in a specific period. Too much competition will dull the excitement, the passion and possibly blunt the killer instinct, taking away all the factors you need to be a winner time and time again.

'It's important to prepare so that you peak for the major events,' says Jeremy Guscott. 'Playing against the best opposition raises aspirations and standards and you want to do well, so you are more alert, more concentrated.'

The more you get used to the feeling of pre-race nerves, that sick empty feeling in your stomach, the more likely it is that in time you will get used to it, handle the pressure and hopefully perform better. Knowing your own ability and how you perform against others sometimes gives you a mental advantage that will help you to perform physically better on the day.

The adrenalin surge you feel before you start is like no other feeling – apart, that is, from winning itself.

After winning it feels like nothing else matters. It doesn't matter how tired you are, for one split second you feel as if all the pain and discomfort has been worth it. You forget all the trauma you have been through. You feel on top of the world. The sheer relief followed by the elation makes the pain a mere blur and a past memory. Some might say it's even better than sex.

The feeling of winning makes you feel as if all the commitment, the hours of hard training, the pain and the sweat were all worthwhile. What you know is that on the day you've competed faster than anybody else in your race.

No one can take that feeling away from you.

ANSWERS TO QUESTIONS

CHAPTER 3

1. 10
2. O Negative
3. 10 pints
4. Decrease
5. 65%
6. Pasta
7. 40%
8. Higher
9 16
10. Both the same
11. 21
12. 60 minutes
13. 2lbs
14. The same, semi-skimmed contains less fat

CHAPTER 4

1. 10lbs
2. 7 hours

3. 70 beats per minute

4. Away

5. 40 mg

6. Microwave oven

7. 60 hours

8. The back of the thigh

9. 75 pints

10. The kidneys

11. 33 vertebrae

12. In the ear – called the stapes or the stirrup

CHAPTER 5

1. B 52 is an American bomber

2. True – they contain vitamin A

3. 4 pints

4. Fluoride

5. 22%

6. Average portion of pilau rice

7. 5–5.3 litres per minute

8. CO_2 – carbon dioxide

9. 35%

10. Greek yogurt

11. 150 calories

12. The liver

CHAPTER 12

1. 5 teaspoons

2. False they contain the same amount of fat and calories

3. 99%

4. Three chocolate digestives

5. 110 calories

6. Plain chocolate

7. 4,100mg

8. The kidneys

9. 4 calories

10. 4 calories

11. 9 calories

12. 200mg

CHAPTER 13

1. 1 cup low-fat milk

2. coconut oil

3. All of the above

4. Meat, poultry and fish

5. Mayonnaise

6. Bananas and potatoes

7. Fish and poultry

8. Meat, poultry, fish and beans

9. A tomato

10. All of the above

11. An apple

12. All of the above

ACKNOWLEDGEMENTS

The authors would like to thank Sally Gunnell and Jeremy Guscott and everybody at Action Time, especially Pat Pearson and Mike Taylor. Thanks also to Rex Hazeldine, fitness consultant to Body Heat and Director of the Centre for Coaching and Recreation, Loughborough University; the Royal Navy Physical Training School; Boxtree Publishers and Carlton UK Television. Finally a special thanks to the Body Heat contestants Kirstie Chapman, Jeremy Tiffen, Cindy Parsons and Simon Amery who shared their training secrets.